PRESCRIPTION FOR SURVIVAL

PRESCRIPTION FOR SURVIVAL

Health and Safety in the Health Service

ALLAN KERR
and
ROGER POOLE

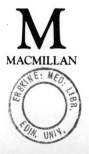

MACMILLAN

First published 1984 by
Higher and Further Education Division
MACMILLAN PUBLISHERS LTD
London and Basingstoke
Companies and representatives throughout the world

British Library Cataloguing in Publication Data
Kerr, Allan
Prescription for survival.
1. Medical care   Great Britain   Safety aspects
I. Title   II. Poole, Roger
363.1'575   RA485
ISBN 0–333–35086–3
ISBN 0–333–35087–1 pbk

Printed in Hong Kong

Contents

Preface

A glimpse of cynicism is likely to cross the face of any union safety rep told that health and safety is an issue taken seriously by health service employers. In fact, they could be forgiven for finding this hard to believe on the evidence before them. Just getting safety advice is a major exercise, as employers cannot or will not provide it. Even books on the subject of health and safety cater mainly for industry. For instance, they do not deal with the problems of lifting and handling of patients or the risks of contracting infectious diseases. Neither do they cater for the needs of community nurses and health visitors who work in the home, which is where most accidents happen.

In the pages which follow we cover most health and safety problems found in the health services. We hope the book will prove useful to all health service workers, particularly union safety reps. It builds on the TUC safety reps' course by providing an introduction to the problems unique to the health services and their control. We also hope that the book kindles a deeper interest in the subject and that some will want to delve deeper by making use of the references on which each chapter is based. Having said all that, administrators and others might read it simply to find out how trade unions view these matters. Of course, we hope they will then do something about them.

We have not catalogued health and safety problems by occupational groups since to do so is to misunderstand the nature of the health services. In hospitals, for instance, a team of people with various skills provide health care in the same workplace; doctors, nurses, porters and physiotherapists might find themselves facing the same health and safety problems while working together on a surgical ward. So we have provided information on the hazards in each workplace as well as on common problems like stress which affect all staff.

Of course, it is a paradox that a service dedicated to caring for the health of the community is at the same time putting the health of its own staff at risk. We hope this book will help, in some measure, to redress this shortcoming by furnishing information which can be used by safety reps to make their workplaces safer.

Woolwich, London, 1983   *A.K.*
         R.P.

Acknowledgements

We are indebted to the Executive Council of the National Union of Public Employees for their support and encouragement in the writing of this book. We are also grateful for having had the opportunity to draw upon the experiences of other trade unions in the Health Service.

Our thanks go to Mike Cunningham and Alan Dalton for reading the first draft and making many helpful comments that have made the final draft readable, though the final outcome, mistakes and all, is our responsibility. A special thanks must go to Pat Pumfrey for showing patience and good humour when typing and retyping the manuscript.

How to Use this Book

Unless you have plenty of time on your hands you might not get round to reading all of this book. We don't expect you to, rather you can pick out the topics relevant to the problems you are dealing with at the time. For instance, before inspecting a ward, you should read the sections on wards, backpain, noise, stress and assaults. For anyone needing more detailed information we suggest using the references which form the basis of each chapter. Finally, at the end of each chapter a checklist is given; it is only a guide and should be tailored to meet local requirements.

1. Why and How Accidents Occur

In 1948 the National Health Service was established, described by many as the greatest triumph of post-war Britain. But it is no longer what its founder, the then Minister of Health, Nye Bevan, intended. Over half of the 2,655 hospitals were built before 1918 and much of its equipment is old and in need of replacement. The conditions staff and patients have to endure are sometimes appalling. A recent article by Bev Gilligan in the *Daily Mirror* (3 February 1983) vividly describes the scene in an outer-London hospital:

> A porter holds an umbrella as an old woman is trundled through a maze of asbestos and plywood huts for an X-ray.
>
> The huts that form the hospital — and too many others in Britain — date from the First and Second World Wars.
>
> Heat from the pipes that stretch across the ward ceilings vanishes rapidly through the felt-covered roofs. In heavy rain, puddles form in the dark, dreary corridors.

To add to the catalogue of problems, most hospitals are faced with staff shortages and constant cash crises. One hospital in the Midlands required £4 million to run its antiquated equipment but the allocation for 1983 was a paltry £80,000. Typical of the problems facing the nursing officer was a sister hysterical with the stress of coping with staff shortages. To save money the medical records officer switched off the heater in her office before going to the toilet.

Against this background it will come as no surprise to learn that safety issues have taken a back seat. Money is simply not made available. The Department of Health and Social Security issued a circular on the setting up of occupational health departments but no money was made available to finance them; health authorities were told cash must come from existing budgets. With hospitals

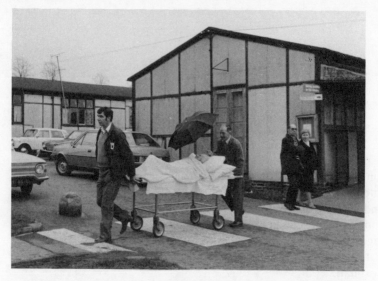

An old woman's journey for an X-ray (courtesy Syndication International Ltd).

crying out for modernisation, hospital wards mothballed because of staff shortages, and patients waiting up to three years for operations, it is pretty obvious that health and safety will get a low priority when it comes to sharing out the health authority budgets. The main problem is a shortage of cash: the government simply does not provide enough money for the running of our health services. As a result the health of patients and staff alike suffers. In fact, one District Management Team (DMT) went as far as to say in their budget proposal for 1978 (quoted in *Hazards Bulletin*, May 1979):

> If pay budgets underspend ... the DMT will continue to make allocations for non-recurring revenue proposals ... the DMT will pay particular attention to the backlog of maintenance work, the replacement of equipment, fire precautions and the implementation of requirements which may result from such statutes as the Health and Safety at Work Act.

Faced with a shortage of cash, the DMT is saying to staff: your wages or your safety! In the rest of this book we look at what this actually means to health service workers.

HOW MANY ACCIDENTS?

Are hospitals safe places to work? The short answer to this question is No. Surprising though it may seem, accident statistics are not available from the Department of Health and Social Security so we have to rely on information gathered by the Health and Safety Executive (HSE) and individual hospitals to know what is happening. We can get some idea of the size of the problem by looking at two surveys of accidents in hospitals. First, the HSE pilot study *Working Conditions in the Medical Service*, published in 1976, gives an analysis of the accidents in one hospital (table 1.1).

Hospital workers in this establishment suffer between one and two dozen accidents every month — the majority of them cuts, bruises and sprains. There were no deaths but there were around three major accidents involving fractures each year. Another survey of accidents in six hospitals with varying specialities ranging from a general hospital to a hospital dealing with orthopaedic specialities and rheumatic and chest conditions had a total of 880 accidents involving hospital workers, again no deaths. But these figures are only a disconnected part of the jigsaw until some form of national reporting is available.

Table 1.1

Total number of reported accidents in one hospital

	1969	1970	1971	1972	1973	1974
Injuries	144	176	233	216	176	235

Prescription for survival

Table 1.2

Accidents according to injury in one hospital

Injuries	1969	1970	1971	1972	1973	1974
Lacerations, abrasions, wounds	56	60	87	71	51	81
Burns	20	13	22	38	26	29
Splinters	4	13	13	8	1	3
Back strain	2	8	17	9	20	19
Other strains, sprains or bruises	44	64	64	65	50	80
Infected wounds	4	2	4	2	2	–
Eye injuries	7	12	17	12	10	1
Ear injuries	–	–	–	–	–	1
Fractures	6	2	1	3	4	1
Head injuries	–	2	8	8	11	10
Electric shock	1	–	–	–	1	–
Total	144	176	233	216	176	235

Of course, simply looking at numbers hides the pain and suffering of these individuals. When we look at the types of injuries we see the extent of the suffering in table 1.2, again taken from the HSE pilot study just mentioned. These figures stress the point we made at the beginning of this section that hospitals are not safe places to work. A few of these injuries may be minor but many, like burns, are very painful and some such as back injuries are disabling and often remain with individuals for most of their working lives. Very rarely do any of these accidents get reported by the press or television. Yet strikes in the health services that might put patients at risk capture the headlines of tabloid newspapers well before anyone is hurt. Just one victim of a dispute merits banner headlines across the front pages of the press. Let us look at some of the accidents to staff not reported by the press.

PERSONAL ACCOUNTS

Jackie

Jackie worked on a hip unit and was expected to lift and turn patients, including an elderly unco-operative and awkward paraplegic patient with the help of only one other nurse. On previous occasions when the patient had been very ill, four nurses had been needed to lift and turn him, but only two nurses were free at the time Jackie was injured. In the past she had hurt her back while lifting patients, and had fully reported these incidents, but the hospital management did nothing about them nor did they warn her about the risks of continuing with this work. With this patient complaints about the difficulties of lifting him were made but ignored. Eventually Jackie got over £8,000 compensation in spite of the fact that management denied liability.

Susan

Back injuries are common among nurses so it is worthwhile looking at what happened to another nurse. Susan was a staff nurse on an orthopaedic ward when the accident occurred. She and a colleague, a nursing auxiliary, were lifting an elderly patient to a sitting position using the traditional lift. Of course, management denied liability and said that she had failed to use the prescribed lifting method she had been taught and had also failed to get help. In fact, she had last undergone training ten years previously which included only an hour's teaching on the lifting and moving of patients. Even the judge hearing her claim for compensation was appalled by this case. He said that management had clearly tolerated nurses lifting in situations where they could injure themselves, and that training on the correct methods of moving and handling patients should have been given, as well as advice on the dangers of moving heavy patients.

Assaults on staff are an increasing problem, particularly in the casualty departments of inner-city hospitals like those of Birmingham, Glasgow, Liverpool and London. Robert's case is typical of the violence occurring on a Saturday night after the pubs close.

Robert

In the early hours of the morning, Robert, an ambulance driver, brought a patient into the casualty department of a London hospital. A youth accompanied by several friends was being abusive to the receptionist when Robert arrived. Several times she asked him to wait outside but he refused. Finally, he said 'Come outside just you and me,' pointing his finger at her. At that point Robert intervened, asking the youth to control his language. Suddenly he pushed Robert, striking him with a head butt, injuring his face. A few minutes later the police arrived to arrest the youth.

WHY DO ACCIDENTS HAPPEN?

Many employers answer this question by blaming the worker. For instance, in their safety booklet *Passport to Safety* the motor company British Leyland wrote: 'Accidents don't just happen, they are caused by your own or someone else's failure, neglect or thoughtlessness.' Perhaps an extreme case, unlikely to be repeated in the health services, but nevertheless an example of the 'careless worker' theory: accidents don't happen because of badly designed machinery, lack of training or supervision, or inadequate systems of work but are the fault of thoughtless workers. Are workers responsible for most accidents at work? Let us look at some typical examples.

Two kitchen workers were off sick, so the rest of the staff had to cope with the extra work. Pat slipped on the floor and broke her leg. Did the accident occur because she was careless? Spillages were not cleaned up as soon as they happened. Was pressure of work to blame? The answer is probably Yes, but we don't think it is that simple. The floor should have been made of a non-slip material to reduce the likelihood of slipping. And management should also have made certain that the kitchen was properly staffed so that all spillages were cleaned up. All too often, workers become ill after exposure to certain cleaning agents. For instance, the combination of ordinary bleach and Harpic produces the toxic gas chlorine which causes burns and can seriously damage the lungs. Should workers use protective clothing and equipment? That might be the employers' solution but we would argue that different cleaning agents should be provided.

Although no two accidents are similar, certain common facts exist. We will look briefly at these.

Training

Susan, whom we met earlier, last underwent training ten years before her accident. Even then she only had one hour's training in lifting and handling patients. Clearly, had she been given both theoretical and practical training in lifting techniques and the use of lifting aids, her accident wouldn't have happened. Indeed, regular refresher training courses would probably have been helpful. All too often, no training is given or it is limited to 'on the job' training. If, however, accidents are to be avoided this isn't any use.

Employers now have an obligation under section 2(2)(c) of the Health and Safety at Work Act to give instruction and training. We consider that to fulfil this requirement basic safety training should be given to all new employees as part of any induction course. In addition, more specialist training may be required for certain jobs. Of course, refresher courses should be available to all staff on a regular basis.

Supervision

Very often accidents could be prevented had the job been properly supervised. For instance, it is doubtful whether Susan would have hurt her back if the ward sister had been around to supervise the lifting of the patient. Clearly, this begs the question: is the supervisor properly trained? A survey done for an HSC working party on the lifting of patients found that some senior nurses were not familiar with the new lifting techniques and did not encourage trainee nurses to follow the lifting principles learnt at training school. Faced with this situation, employers must make sure not only that jobs are correctly supervised but also that supervisors are trained where safety is concerned. Again, employers actually have a legal duty under the Health and Safety at Work Act to provide adequate supervision.

Information

Following a visit from an inspector, an improvement notice was served on a hospital for failing to provide written instructions on the safe working procedures to be followed when handling materials containing asbestos. This case makes the point that employers don't always give workers sufficient information about the dangers of their work and the safe working practices which ought to be followed, despite the requirement under section 2(2)(c) of the Health and Safety at Work Act to provide advice. Such neglect is more than simply breaking the law: it puts workers' lives at risk.

Machine Design

Machines are very often designed to do a specific job without attention being paid to the operator's safety. We can think of several examples:

- the rotating blade of a waste disposal unit in the kitchens not effectively guarded;
- the transmission machinery of a washing machine in the laundry

not securely fenced; similarly, the chain and sprocket drive to the rollers of a squeeze unit not properly fenced;
- the blade of a metal-cutting guillotine not securely fenced.

Although the machines had guards, they obviously did not protect workers from the dangerous moving parts. In most cases they could be removed without stopping the machines operating. So, as long as this state of affairs continues, accidents are going to happen.

Systems of Work

In the words of the HSE,

> Systems of work means the way in which the work is organised and includes, for example, the layout of the workplace, the order in which jobs are carried out, or special precautions that have to be taken before carrying out certain hazardous tasks. This duty therefore means that, for example, a machine itself, and the way it is operated, must both be safe. (From: *A Guide to the HSW Act*, Health and Safety Series booklet HS(R)6, obtainable from HMSO.)

Put simply, it means employers must see that jobs are done in the safest possible way. Let us look at some examples.
- In one hospital the arrangements for entering confined spaces in the sewage plant were inadequate. A safe system of work was needed which included using a safety harness, gas testing equipment and breathing apparatus.
- Another example involved the removal of asbestos lagging by maintenance staff. If the work had gone ahead as planned the workers would have been exposed to loose asbestos fibres. Instead it was stopped until a safe system of work could be devised to protect them. Incidents of this kind are common, suggesting that unless employers give some thought to how the work is actually done, bearing safety in mind, accidents and ill health will continue to dog workers.

There are obviously other factors which contribute to the causes of accidents and we look at these in other chapters.

WHY JOIN A UNION?

Throughout this book we argue that trade unions are the most effective means of getting healthier and safer working conditions. In this section we look at why you should join a trade union and how it can help improve your working conditions. We begin by looking at why individuals are not as successful as unions in achieving things.

The Worker

Since the beginning of the last century workers have been struggling to get better wages and greater job security as well as improved working conditions. There is an obvious conflict of interest between the employer and workers over all these issues. The employer will want to keep costs as low as possible, which in practice means spending as little as possible on the workplace, not to mention wages. From the worker's point of view, it means a continuous fight to get the employer to provide a living wage and a reasonable working environment.

In this struggle, workers quickly learn that individuals cannot win on their own. Employers brand anyone who complains about wages, job losses or working conditions a 'trouble-maker', and it is not very long before they are shown the hospital gate. History has shown that the only defence against being victimised is combining together. The slogan 'united we stand, divided we fall' probably best sums up this principle. Employers are more likely to pick a fight with an individual than with the whole workforce: there's safety in numbers.

The Union

Although arguing for better wages and service conditions has been the main preoccupation for unions, it is not the only interest.

Health and safety has always been on the shopping list. For all that, it must be said that it has had a much lower priority than other aims. However, union interest in this matter has taken on a new lease of life since the Safety Representatives Regulations came into operation in 1978. One example is the fight to ban the

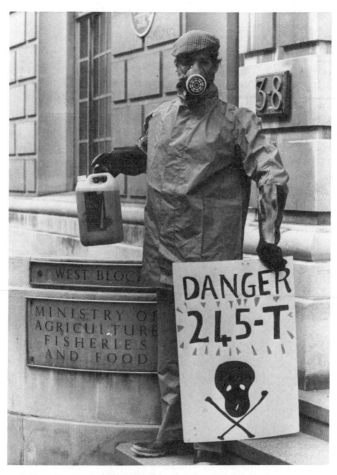

Dumping the weedkiller 2, 4, 5-T on the steps of the Ministry of Agriculture as part of the TGWU campaign to have it banned (courtesy Press Association Ltd).

weedkiller 2,4,5-T. This is linked with cancer, heart disease, miscarriages and birth defects. Despite all the evidence the government said there is no reason why 2,4,5-T should be banned. Not satisfied with this response, several unions got employers to withdraw it from use. The farmworkers' union, now part of the Transport and General Workers Union, went further and organised a campaign to have the chemical banned. Many employers reacted by withdrawing it despite government assurances over its safety.

The Law

All too often, it is said that the law protects workers' welfare by providing certain minimum health and safety standards which an employer must comply with. However, at the same time the law takes into account what it is reasonable for that employer to do. Very often there is a difference of opinion over this point which may end up in court. But history shows that judgments are more often in favour of employers. And to make matters worse, the law is not always watertight, which allows employers to find loopholes to their advantage. So where does this leave workers if they cannot rely on the law? The answer is: using the union to safeguard their own health and safety by improving working conditions.

Safety Representatives

Since 1978 unions have had the right to appoint safety representatives in the workplace to improve working conditions. In Chapter 8 we look in detail at their role, which can be summarised as:

- to inspect the workplace every three months;
- to inspect the site of a dangerous occurrence or notifiable accident;
- to inspect the workplace after a notifiable disease has been contracted;
- to investigate potential hazards and accident sites;
- to inspect certain documents and be given certain information by their employer;
- to receive information from inspectors;

- to investigate complaints by members.

It is important to remember, however, that only recognised trade unions have been given the right to appoint safety representatives. In this context, a recognised union is one which negotiates with the employer over wages and conditions of service on behalf of the workforce. So the law only gives workers who belong to a recognised union the right to appoint safety representatives.

Using the Union

As we say earlier, organising for better wages and working conditions has been the major function of unions. That experience can be put to good use in the struggle to achieve improvements in the workplace. In particular, the Union can help workers by exchanging information, by pursuing its members' claims for compensation, and by pressing for changes in the law.

Exchanging Information

Safety representatives need to combat lack of interest in health and safety and to build support for their own activities. This is a continuous headache for them. However, the existing structures of the union can be used. For instance, branch meetings can have a place on the agenda for safety issues, so that members can raise problems and even decide on the demands for the safety representative to approach management with. Equally, full use can be made of the union's printing facilities to produce safety broadsheets or leaflets. Indeed, safety representatives may even want to print posters.

Some unions provide safety reps with information about hazards and other technical matters. In fact, nearly all health service unions issue handbooks for their safety reps with commentaries on the Health and Safety at Work Act as well as the Safety Representatives and Safety Committees Regulations. Although the extent of the service varies, most unions have staff to give advice and support to safety reps. In addition to the numerous occupational health and safety guides, several unions publish hazard warning sheets. For instance, ASTMS issue *Health and Safety*

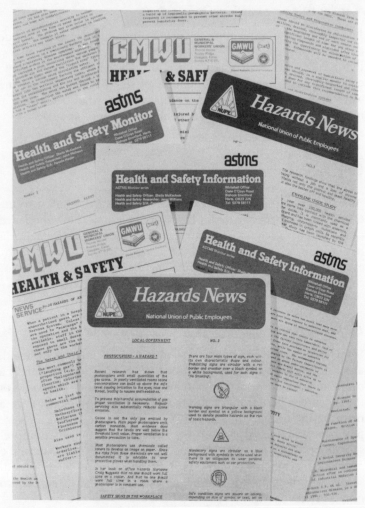

Unions' hazard warning sheets.

Monitor dealing with specific hazards like Legionnaires disease. Of course, these services are available only to union members.

Compensation

One of the traditional roles of the union is the provision of legal services to get members compensation whenever they suffer an accident or illness at work. In spite of the emphasis on prevention there is still a need for this service. Jackie, mentioned earlier, got over £8,000 compensation for a back injury after her union took her case to court.

Improving the Law

Although the law lays down standards with which employers must comply there are certain weaknesses. First, it only sets minimum standards which are often unsatisfactory. It is left to the union to improve on these through collective bargaining and by organising campaigns to change the law. A recent example is the campaign to tighten the laws on asbestos led by the GMBATU. Second, the law is interpreted by judges who are, as we said earlier, more likely to find in favour of the employer. Furthermore, employers can afford lawyers to find ways round the law. Faced with this situation, the union can either deal with the problem through collective bargaining using industrial action as coercion or again by campaigning to have the loopholes in the law removed.

To sum up, the union can help by:

- appointing safety reps;
- co-ordinating workplace action to improve conditions;
- campaigning for effective safety laws.

REFERENCES

Health and Safety Executive (1976). *Pilot Study—Working Conditions in the Medical Services*.

Accidents. *Hazards Bulletin No.8*, Oct. 1977. British Society for Social Responsibility in Science, PO Box 148, Sheffield S1 1FB.

J.A. Lunn (1976). *The Health of Staff in Hospitals*, Heinemann Medical Books, London, ch.10.

Bedford General Hospital, Occupational Health Service (1975). *7th and Final Report*, North Bedfordshire Health Authority, Bedford.

R.G. Lee (1979). Health and safety in hospitals, *Med. Sci. Law*, **19**, No.2.

Working Group on Lifting of Patients in the Health Service (1982). *Report*. A private communication to the Health Services Advisory Committee of the Health and Safety Commission.

2. Where Accidents Happen

Throughout this book, we say that nearly all accidents, ill health and diseases are avoidable. The struggle for workers is to make the workplace safer, basically by doing two things; first, finding out what the health and safety problems are and, second, getting their employer to do something about them. So in this chapter we set out to look at the different workplaces in a hospital, to show what dangers exist and to point out how to overcome them. Instead of looking at the risks by occupation, we have chosen to do it by workplace simply because people in different jobs may all find themselves working in the same place facing the same dangers. For example, on a busy morning you will probably find nurses, porters, doctors, ward orderlies and maybe even laboratory technicians working in a hospital ward. Using this workplace approach, safety reps should be able to spot hazards and arm themselves with some basic knowledge on how to deal with them.

Clearly, getting the employer to actually do something about the hazards is more difficult, especially when the government department holding the purse-strings is the DHSS. Most health authorities will plead poverty, or, to put it another way, will say the proposals are just too costly. But don't let this parsimonious attitude stop you. As we explain in more detail later on, section 2 of the Health and Safety at Work Act can be used to get health authorities to actually do something about health and safety matters. Of course, you will have the problem of what is 'reasonably practicable' for them to do, and, in the final analysis, industrial action may be the only way to get money spent on health and safety.

Having set the scene, we now look in detail at the different workplaces in a hospital.

KITCHENS

All too often, working in a hospital kitchen is unpleasant and dangerous. In the HSE pilot study, *Working Conditions in the Health Service*, kitchens were responsible for 12 per cent of all staff accidents. Cuts are a major source of injury, knives and can openers being the main culprits. Other injuries include burns and scalds from handling hot pans and cooking with fat. And high temperatures in summer sometimes make working in the kitchens almost unbearable.

Common Risks and their Controls

Detergents and other cleaning products.   Dishwashers may suffer from dermatitis because they are allergic to certain detergents. Contact with cleaning agents for floors, work surfaces and cooking equipment can have similar results. In this situation the answer is to use less irritating cleaning products or make use of protective clothing like rubber gloves with cotton liners. Management should also give advice on skin care.

Floors.   Wet or greasy floors, usually the result of spillages or condensation, can cause nasty accidents. Aisles cluttered with cables, food and kitchen utensils are a frequent problem.

Spillages ought to be cleared as soon as they occur, and adequate ventilation usually overcomes condensation problems. Avoid wet floors and insist upon the use of non-slip polish. Remove all obstructions from the aisles.

Fat fryers, ovens and grills.   Where there is an accumulation of grease, fires can occur.

Essentially, following good housekeeping principles and ensuring that these appliances are kept free of grease will usually prevent fires breaking out.

Chip pan fires can be avoided by simply keeping the oil level well below the top of deep fat fryers.

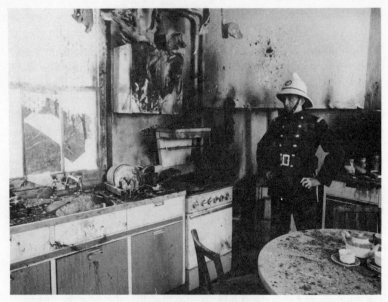

**After a chip pan fire
(courtesy London Fire Brigade).**

Nevertheless, the risk of fat fires cannot be totally eliminated, so fire-extinguishers compatible with fat should be readily available. Foam fire-extinguishers are the most suitable, and common sense tells you not to locate them too near the potential source of fire. Fire blankets made from heat-resistant leather are best for chip pan fires. It is also worthwhile insisting upon training in the use of all equipment.

Ovens, pipes, pots, pans and stoves.   Burns and scalds are the most serious hazard here. Simple precautions can prevent these injuries happening. Insist upon all pipes being properly insulated with non-asbestos material and use oven gloves or cloths to lift hot pans and dishes.

Steam is a common cause of burns in the kitchen. All equipment using it must be regularly serviced to prevent leaks, particularly pressure cookers.

Lighting.   Poor lighting can be a persistent problem but one which is readily overcome by regularly cleaning all windows and keeping them free from all obstruction. All broken or missing bulbs or tubes should be replaced immediately. Of course, the amount of lighting depends very much on the type of work being done. In kitchens 500–600 lux is adequate. If, however, the lighting is still unsatisfactory, advice should be sought from a lighting expert.

Temperature   At the beginning of this section we refer to the problems of working in a hot environment, and point out that more accidents happen when the temperature rises.

The immediate solution to this problem, especially in summer, is for the staff to be given adequate breaks. However, in the long term, the kitchen must be designed to ensure adequate ventilation. See Chapter 5 for further advice on this problem.

Food products.   Earlier we referred to the risk of dermatitis when handling cleaning agents. Certain foodstuffs are also sensitising agents, causing allergic reactions in some people handling them; these can include flour, cinnamon and vanilla.

Anyone experiencing this should get help from the local-authority environmental health officer in identifying those substances responsible and avoid contact with them by using safe-handling procedure. If this proves unsatisfactory a job change within the hospital is the answer.

Kitchen environment.   Stress can occur particularly during rushed meal times. In this situation management must review their time-tabling to minimise pressure as well as providing sufficient staff to match the workload.

Catering Equipment

In this part we examine some of the common risks of working with specialist kitchen equipment, and how to control them.

Can openers.   Worn blades are the main cause of accidents, so arrange to have them replaced regularly.

Dishwashing machines.   Accidents are most likely to happen if someone removes the inspection cover or looks inside when the machine is operating. The rule here is never to open the inspection cover or look inside while the machine is working. Of course, it is much better to fit a lock which comes into operation while the machine is operating. As well as these precautions, make sure that the safety screens are in position at each end and in good condition.

Fat fryers.   Burns are the most common injury and are caused by hot fat. Before frying check to see that there is sufficient fat to cover the thermostat. Lower the food slowly into the hot fat using appropriate cooking utensils. Since the risk of fire is always present, don't leave the fryer unattended while cooking.

Knives.   Cuts, usually minor, though often requiring stitches, do occur. To reduce the likelihood of an accident knives should be:

- kept in a designated storage area when not in use with the blades not exposed;
- kept sharpened and in good condition;
- carried with the point downwards;
- washed separately and never left in washing water;
- used with a cutting board or other firm surface when cutting, dicing or chopping.

Mincers.   Accidents can happen when the machine is being cleaned or when the feed is operated by hand. Before cleaning a mincer, or in fact any electric machinery, disconnect the power supply. Never operate the feed by hand; always use a plunger.

Potato peelers.   The main causes of accidents here are peering too close to the bowl or placing hands in it when the machine is operating. To make sure that you avoid cuts or eye injuries just don't peer too close or put your hands in the bowl when it is in use.

Potato chippers.   Accidents will not happen as long as you:

- always feed the chipper by using a plunger;
- make sure that the blade guard is in position before using the machine;
- switch off the power before clearing a blockage.

Slicing machine. This machine is dangerous and should be operated only with the blade guard in position. Don't push the food towards the blade by hand; use the 'last slice' method.

LABORATORIES

In a survey of hospital laboratories reported in the *Journal of the Society of Occupational Medicine* in 1977, none were found to satisfy the minimum standards set down in law. The survey showed shortcomings in ventilation, cleanliness, illumination, storage of chemicals, fire precautions and the use and maintenance of mechanical equipment. But most disconcerting was the failure on the part of the commissioning team responsible for the design specification to take into account health and safety needs. One hospital went as far as placing laboratories containing toxic, infectious and fire hazards on the first floor of a multi-storey building.

In several of the laboratories, dangerous toxic and corrosive chemicals were stored on shelves without rails or curving lips, gas cylinders were not adequately secured in an upright position, and fire exits were blocked, many with highly flammable material. Simple design errors were found such as bad lighting. Quite often artificial lighting was incorrectly positioned or white bench surfaces caused glare from reflected sunlight.

Even basic health and safety standards were flouted. Poor standards of cleanliness and decoration were often apparent. This was most noticeable in the newest and largest of the hospitals in the survey. And in some cases active steps had not been taken to stop staff smoking and eating food in the laboratories.

Other horror stories include the case of a chemical pathology laboratory in a well-known medical school where benzene, a common carcinogenic, was found on open shelves. What makes this nearly unbelievable is that a safer chemical, toluene, was readily available and could certainly have been used as a substitute.

Common Risks and their Controls

In this section we have chosen not to give more than basic health and safety advice, because of the numerous and varied kinds of work done by laboratory staff. But each health service establishment where laboratories are sited should give detailed guidance on the procedures to be followed in them.

Biological agents

Staff are exposed to the risk of infection from handling and disposing of contaminated blood, urine, faeces, sputum or organs. Among the measures that can be taken to reduce the likelihood of infection are:

- knowledge about the dangers of these agents and how to recognise symptoms of exposure;
- familiarity with the safe-handling and disposal procedures;
- understanding of the use of protective clothing and equipment;
- availability and use of antidotes.

Two basic rules that should *not* be broken are:

- never pipette by mouth;
- never eat, drink or smoke in the laboratory, or store food in laboratory refrigerators.

Chemicals

Toxic substances can enter the body through different routes: the skin, lungs, or digestive system. Therefore, safety reps need to know something about these when deciding on the best way to prevent them happening.

Skin.   On contacting the skin some chemicals:

- cause inflammation of the skin (dermatitis);
- permeate through the skin into the bloodstream;
- cause a reaction by the body against them after frequent contact (sensitisation).

Lungs.   Dusts, gases and vapours can be inhaled, causing irritation and inflammation of the lungs.

Digestive system. Swallowing chemicals can happen if workers eat, drink or smoke in their presence.

Thus any precautions must take into account the way a chemical is likely to enter the body. For instance, formaldehyde irritates the skin and lungs, so steps need to be taken to prevent both contact with the skin and airborne contamination.

As well as establishing how chemicals enter the body, safety reps need to know the effect they can have. Reactions can fall into two groups, acute and chronic. In cases where the body reacts immediately to exposure, as with excessive consumption of alcohol, the effect is acute. By contrast, chronic effects, like alcoholism, came about from repeated exposure to low doses of chemicals. Normally, the symptoms go unnoticed since their onset is gradual. A knowledge of the differences between acute and chronic effects is required because the precautions for controlling them may vary. But it also has to be remembered that quite often the chronic effects are not known. So measures for controlling acute effects may subsequently prove to be unsatisfactory for controlling chronic effects.

Faced with these problems, safety reps should start from the assumption that no chemical found in the laboratory is safe or harmless. So make sure there are:

- safe disposal, handling and storage procedures;
- spill procedures;
- clear warning labels on all chemicals and a scheme to replace them when they become unreadable;

and that there is:

- information about the hazards, exposure symptoms and precautions;
- the installation of exhaust ventilation, particularly local exhaust or fume hoods;
- provision of protective clothing and equipment. But this should be regarded as only a back-up and not a first line of defence.

No attempt has been made to put these points in any order of priority. All of them should be kept in mind.

Where a chemical is known to be highly dangerous try to find an alternative substance. But beware of new chemicals because they may have unknown hazards. If substitution is not possible, the chemical should be used in an enclosed system with special arrangements for storage. Among laboratory chemicals known to be highly dangerous are a group of known or suspected carcinogenics: benzidine, ortho-tolidine, diamino-benzidine, benzene, bis-chloromethyl, ether, mustine hydrochloride and immune-suppressive drugs. Benzidine is a prohibited substance and should not be handled.

With some chemicals there is a risk of an explosion or fire. This risk can be minimised by ensuring the work area is free of potential ignition sources except bunsen burners. All flammable liquids should be stored in specially designed safety containers. Not all fires and explosions are caused by ignition sources; some occur as a result of chemical reactions, so everyone should be familiar with the procedure to be followed in the event of one of these incidents.

Laboratory equipment

Users of laboratory equipment should keep two things in mind. First, they should insist on being given training in the use of all equipment, in how to recognise malfunctions and in emergency procedures. Second, they should insist on regular inspections and maintenance by qualified technicians.

In particular:

- With centrifuges, breakages can occur, exposing the operator to broken glass and contaminated droplets. After a breakage, allow time for the droplets to settle before autoclaving all the parts. Make certain suitable protective clothing is worn when clearing up. Broken glass will not be such a serious problem as long as there are locks on the centrifuge head.
- Poor maintenance of autoclaves often allows steam to escape; this emphasises the importance of regular maintenance.

Compressed-gas cylinders

Oxygen, hydrogen, carbon dioxide and many other gases find a wide range of uses in hospitals. The obvious danger here is of explosions followed by fire, but a few simple precautions can reduce it. Insist on:

- all cylinders being stored and secured in an upright position;
- valve protection caps being fastened when not in use;
- all cylinders being clearly marked;
- showers and protective clothing being available for those handling or working with compressed gases.

Several codes of practice on safe working procedures are available and should be kept for reference in the laboratory. For example, the Code of Practice for the Prevention of Infection in Clinical Laboratories and Post-Mortem Rooms, known also as the Howie Code.

LAUNDRIES

Visiting the local launderette on a hot summer's day is an unpleasant experience. The heat inside quickly tires one, leaving a feeling of lethargy and debility. But for laundry staff this is merely one of the many potential hazards that they face. Backpain through heavy lifting, dermatitis from frequent contact with detergents and accidents involving machinery are all part of the catalogue of risks that daily confronts them. In fact, laundries have been recognised as dangerous places to work and were incorporated in the Factories Act 1961.

Common Hazards and their Controls

Floors. Wet floors are a major cause of accidents and should be avoided as much as possible. If, however, floors are continually wet, management should improve the draining and provide non-slip flooring. Serious leg injuries have occurred where floor drainage channels have not been adequately covered and maintained.

Detergents. Continuous immersion in hot water and the handling of a variety of detergents can cause dermatitis. To avoid this problem either use less irritating detergent or use protective clothing including rubber gloves with cotton liners.

Linen. Laundry staff are exposed to the risk of infection from contaminated clothing or bed linen, particularly from isolation wards. You must insist upon the introduction of safe-handling procedures and that all laundry bags are clearly labelled to indicate the status of the infection.

Needles, knives and other surgical instruments left in soiled linen cause cuts and puncture wounds. As well as handling with care, laundry staff should wear heavy gloves. But constant reminders should be issued to staff, especially doctors, warning them not to leave 'sharps' in clothing or bed linen.

In a letter to the medical journal *The Lancet* (5 June 1982), a laundry manageress describes some of the health risks to staff:

350 items were collected of 48 different types with an estimated replacement cost of £600–£700. Examples are as follows:

Hazards, potentially infectious	*Number*	
Incontinence pads	21	
Soiled dressings	2	(large bags)
Urinals (contents mixed with laundry)	8	
Bedpans (contents mixed with laundry)	9	
Colostomy bags (full)	3	
Hazardous, potentially injurious		
Hypodermic needles	15	
Scalpel and razor blades (used)	2	
Scissors	3	

[Consider] the health risk to the staff. So far only minor cuts have been reported but it must be only a matter of time before a case of hepatitis B or similar infection is identified in a laundry worker as being caused by one of these contaminated articles, especially since the contents of bedpans and urinals convert ordinary items to soiled....

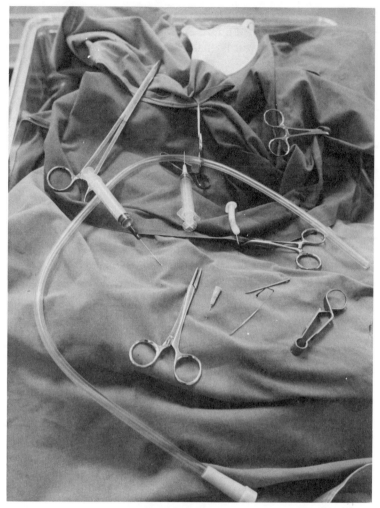

Laundry, some of the safety hazards facing workers (courtesy A. Nicola).

The items have been displayed in the occupational health department and photographed and have been demonstrated to doctors, nurses and administrators, who have expressed horror.

Machinery. According to the International Labour Organisation, crushed or trapped limbs, entangled hair and electric shocks are a few of the hazards that confront staff using specialised laundry equipment.

Standing. A great deal of laundry work involves standing and for some people this can aggravate varicose veins and cause swelling of the feet and ankles. Overcoming this problem can involve:

- frequent rest periods to avoid fatigue;
- job rotation where standing is essential;
- job review to minimise the amount of standing.

Ventilation. At the beginning of this section we mention the problem of high temperatures and heat stress. If ventilation is poor this can give rise to high temperatures and excessive humidity. In this hot and humid atmosphere, staff readily become tired and weak, exhibiting the general symptoms of heat stress.

Clearly, the only satisfactory method of dealing with this problem is to make certain that there is adequate ventilation (see Chapter 5). If, however, this is not immediately possible then steps should be taken to introduce job rotation so that the amount of time spent working in these conditions is kept to a minimum. Similarly, frequent rest periods will reduce the likelihood of heat fatigue.

Noise. See Chapter 5.

OPERATING SUITES

Waste Anaesthetic Gases

In 1842 an American doctor first gave ether as an anaesthetic to a patient. Since then various combinations of anaesthetic gases like halothane, nitrous oxide and oxygen have been used in surgical operations. And it is nearly a hundred years since the first report that staff working in operating rooms could become ill as a result of exposure to anaesthetic gases. But greater attention to these risks has only been paid in the last fifteen years even though there were other reports of the dangers.

A typical combination of anaesthetic gases would be 70 per cent nitrous oxide, 26 to 29 per cent oxygen and 1 to 4 per cent halothane, although occasionally ether or trichloro-ethylene are substituted for halothane. Normally, this mixture is administered through a face mask, forced ventilation or through an instrument known as an endotracheal tube. For those administering the anaesthetic, the risks come from:

- gas leaks in equipment;
- breathing of the patient, since most of the original anaesthetic mixture is given off to the atmosphere of the operating theatre.

Waste gases of this kind are found in rooms other than the operating theatre. In particular, they are found in delivery rooms, post-operative recovery rooms and certain diagnostic areas.

Waste anaesthetic gases may cause serious health risks, in particular spontaneous abortion, cancer and damage to the nervous system. Other possible health hazards include liver and kidney disease, and the risk of congenital abnormalities in children of people exposed to these gases. We now look at each of these in turn.

Spontaneous abortions

Despite the fact that many scientific studies of this problem can be criticised, there definitely appears to be a higher risk of spontaneous abortion among women exposed to anaesthetic gases. In a Danish study, scientists found that spontaneous abortion among these women is twice as high as among women in other groups. Other studies have also shown that there is a higher risk of malformation among children born by women exposed to anaesthetic gases during pregnancy.

Cancer

There is a rising tide of evidence to suggest that anaesthetic gases act as a cancer-inducing agent. Basically, there are broad similarities between some known human cancer agents and several of the anaesthetic gases now in use. Also, some anaesthetic compounds can turn into chemical cancer-agents in certain situations. A large American study found that women, not men, exposed to anaesthetic gases have a greater likelihood of contracting cancer, especially leukaemia and lymphoma. A recent English study also suggests a higher cancer risk among anaesthetic staff.

Central nervous system

Both animal and human experiments have shown that exposure to anaesthetic gases can affect the central nervous system. Some evidence exists to suggest that the performance of individuals can be impaired after exposure to anaesthetic gases. Further evidence also exists to show that neurologic disorders can occur after prolonged exposure to nitrous oxide. In fact, one study showed that two dentists suffered neurological disorders after working in poorly ventilated offices. It must be said, however, that no studies have been done on the long-term effects of exposure to waste anaesthetic gases on the central nervous system.

Other effects

Some scientists believe liver and kidney damage may occur as a consequence of exposure to these gases but no evidence exists at the moment to suggest that bone marrow may be affected.

To sum up we may conclude that there is a risk of:

- miscarriages (spontaneous abortion);
- birth defects (congenital malformations).

To a lesser extent there is a danger of:

- kidney and liver disease;
- damage to the central nervous system;
- cancers like leukaemia and lymphoma.

What can be done about it?

Dealing with waste anaesthetic gases is a simple business but it does cost money. Back in 1976 the DHSS issued a circular recommending that 'pollution levels should be reduced as far as is practicably possible,' and information was given about suitable scavenging systems. But, despite the fact that the DHSS acknowledged the need for these systems, no extra money was made available. According to ASTMS the result was that only 33 per cent of operating theatres had scavenging systems in 1978. Clearly, waste anaesthetic gases are a serious health hazard, so what can be done if the DHSS will not help?

In fact there is a lot you can do:

- Make certain there is early reporting of pregnancy among operating theatre staff and the allocation of alternative jobs for at least the first three months of pregnancy.
- See that there is a minimum airflow of 2 cubic feet per minute per square foot of floor area (2 cubic metres per minute per square metre) to guarantee ventilation and demand the installation of scavenging systems. Further information on ventilation standards is given in Guidance Note EH22 from the Health and Safety Executive.
- Insist on the regular monitoring of anaesthetic gas levels and effectiveness of ventilation. If there is any doubt ask the HSE local office to monitor the levels for you.
- According to the National Institute of Occupational Safety and Health, there is no safe level of exposure to the halogenated anaesthetic agents, but it recommends that exposure be controlled to around levels of 2 p.p.m., and for nitrous oxide 25 p.p.m. But in Denmark the threshold limit value (TLV) for halothane has been put at 1 p.p.m. These are the levels of exposure to keep in mind that are relatively safe.

Other Hazards and their Control

Instrument sterilisation. A study of sterilising staff in Finnish hospitals suggests that exposure to ethylene oxide, a liquid used for the chemical sterilisation of instruments, may carry a risk of spontaneous abortion. Researchers found that where staff were concerned in sterilising procedures during their pregnancy the frequency for spontaneous abortion was 16.7 per cent compared with 5.6 per cent for non-exposed pregnancies. Interestingly enough, this effect was not observed for the other sterilising chemicals, formaldehyde and gluteraldehyde. However, the researchers add a note of caution to their findings: 'As studies of spontaneous abortions are inherently complex and difficult to control for, confirmation of the results is urgently needed so that the staff concerned in sterilising procedures can be protected.'

Nevertheless, we would argue that all pregnant sterilising staff should be kept away from ethylene oxide until it is shown to be safe.

Cleaning agents for scrubs. Clearly, there is a risk of dermatitis, so where skin irritation occurs insist on less sensitising cleaning agents and advice on skin care. Also, if appropriate, use protective gloves with cotton liners.

Instrument cleaning. Some germicidal disinfectants like stericol can act as sensitising agents, so causing dermatitis. In addition to the advice given above, all containers should be labelled to identify the disinfectants, hazards and precautions.

Instruments. Careless disposal of surgical blades and needles causes cuts and puncture wounds. To deal with them, a scheme should be initiated to keep a check on all surgical equipment so that they are not disposed of in linen and other materials handled by staff. Also, staff should insist upon designated containers for the disposal of these instruments.

Portable X-ray equipment. See section on radiology.

Stress. See Chapter 6.

Electrical machinery and equipment. With further cuts in health service budgets there is an increasing trend to 'do-it-yourself' repairs, which only too often are the cause of electric shocks. This is a particularly dangerous practice, so staff should insist on regular inspections and maintenance by qualified staff.

PHARMACY

Pharmacies have less accidents than other hospital departments. That said, those working in the pharmacy handle a vast number of dangerous chemicals which clearly put their health at risk. As we argue throughout this book, the onus is on the employer to see that hazards are eliminated and advice is available on safe-handling procedures. So insist on full information being made available about the dangers of all chemicals and other products in use. See the section 'Laboratories' for some of the points to watch out for. Also, see under 'Community Nurses' in Chapter 3 for the dangers of cytotoxic drugs.

RADIOLOGY

Since the turn of the century there has been a great increase in the use of radiation in the treatment of patients. Generally, most people associate it with hospital X-ray departments but now radiation is widely used in the treatment of cancer and other malignant diseases. In particular, two new fields of medicine have sprung up, radiotherapy and nuclear medicine, both of which use radiation extensively. In fact, some eighty hospitals or so now have radiotherapy facilities and about four hundred regularly use radioactive substances. Obviously, the greatest risk to staff in this work is exposure to radiation. In this section we look at the hazards that non-ionising and ionising radiation pose to them.

Non-ionising Radiation

Radiation is either ionising or non-ionising. Ionising radiation can easily break the bonds between the very atoms of matter that is subjected to it, whereas non-ionising radiation cannot. In this sense, non-ionising radiation is less potentially hazardous, but it must still be treated with caution.

Non-ionising radiation consists entirely of different kinds of what we call electromagnetic waves: radio waves, including micro-waves, infra-red waves, light and ultra-violet waves. These differ from each other on the basis of their frequency and wavelength. The waves are similar to those made when a stone is thrown into a pond. A succession of circular waves originate from the point where the stone falls and spread out until they reach the pond's edge. Here the wavelength is the distance from the crest of one wave to that of the next and the frequency is the number of waves that die out at the pond's edge in a second. Of the different forms of non-ionising radiation, the lowest-frequency waves are radio waves, next come infra-red waves, then light waves, followed by ultra-violet waves.

We now look at some of the risks of working with this type of radiation. Visible light is not listed, as we can safely say that it does not damage the body. It does cause problems where there is either too much or too little of it, of course, but where this happens we have dealt with it under 'Lighting'.

Ultra-violet radiation (UV)

Effects on skin.   These are twofold: acute effects experienced within a few hours of exposure and chronic effects which may not show up for several years. Most people will recognise the acute effects as sunburn. This is easily seen as a reddening of the skin caused mainly by radiation of wavelengths shorter than 315 nm. The severity of this effect very much depends on the duration and intensity of the exposure. Chronic effects appearing after repeated exposure include premature skin ageing and skin cancer. Again, the wavelengths responsible are below 315 nm. So far, no cases of skin cancer due to occupational exposure have been reported.

Effects on eyes.   Excessive exposure can cause a very painful condition commonly called 'eye flash' or 'arc eye'. The symptoms are pain, something like grit in the eyes and an aversion to light. These appear a few hours after exposure and seldom last more than 36 hours. The most damaging effects are produced at a wavelength of 270 nm.

Protection against over-exposure.   The National Radiological Protection Board recommend the following precautions:

- *Hazard warning*. All staff using the ultra-violet radiation should be informed of the hazards.
- *Warning signs and lights*. Hazard warning signs should be put up to indicate the existence of ultra-violet radiation. Warning lights should be used to show when the equipment is in use.
- *Distance*. Users should keep as far away as possible from the source.

- *Exposure time*. Clearly, exposure time should be kept to an absolute minimum. The National Institute for Occupational Safety and Health (NIOSH) suggests the following maximum exposures:

Wavelength range 400–315 nm
1. The total radiation falling on unprotected eyes and skin for periods of greater than 1,000 seconds should not exceed 10 watts per square metre ($W\ m^{-2}$).
2. The total radiation exposure on unprotected eyes and skin for periods of less than 1,000 seconds should not exceed 10^4 joules per square metre ($J\ m^{-2}$).

Wavelength range 315–200 nm
The total radiation exposure on unprotected eyes and skin should not exceed, within any 8-hour period:

Wavelength	*Maximum permissible exposure*
(nm)	*($J\ m^{-2}$)*
200	1,000
250	70
300	100

Note: We do not give the complete table, only some sample wavelengths. Calculating exposure times is difficult: if there is any doubt call the HSE Inspectorate.

- *Maintenance work*. Always disconnect the power supply before doing any work.
- *Containment*. To prevent indiscriminate radiation into the workplace, either the source should be contained within a sealed housing or, where the exposure process takes place outside the source housing, a screened area should be provided.
- *Interlocks*. These should be fitted to the source housing.
- *Reflections*. To reduce reflected radiation, surfaces should be painted in a dark, matt colour.

- *Personal protection.* As an additional precaution protective clothing should be worn. Backs of hands, forearms, face and neck are most at risk.
- *Protection of the eyes.* Goggles, spectacles or face shields which absorb ultra-violet radiation should be worn wherever there is a potential risk of eye damage.

Ozone danger.　The interaction of ultra-violet radiation with air forms a dangerous gas, ozone. At concentrations of 0.1 parts per million, ozone causes smarting of the eyes and a feeling of discomfort in the nose and throat. At exposures of higher than 1 part per million, ozone causes convulsions and loss of consciousness. However, the presence of the gas is easily detectable by its characteristic, penetrating odour. To avoid the hazard of ozone, make sure there is adequate ventilation. Very intense short-wavelength sources may need an extraction system to remove the ozone.

Infra-red radiation (IR)

Again, over-exposure causes a condition similar to sunburn, and in certain circumstances can burn the eyelids and cause cataracts. This is most likely to happen where heat-therapy treatment is being given. The precautions, excluding the exposure times, are broadly similar to those with ultra-violet radiation.

Microwaves

Exposure to microwaves may occur during diathermy, the modern way of cauterising blood vessels in an operation. But evidence about their harmful effects is conflicting so, to be on the safe side, continuous exposure must not exceed 10 milliwatts per cubic centimetre $(mW\,cm^{-3})$. If, also, there is any doubt about the safety of this apparatus get advice from the local health and safety inspector.

Ionising Radiation

Because all ionising radiation can break the bonds between the very atoms that make up all matter, it can be harmful to living things; in humans it can cause cancer and genetic damage. In fact, the lethal effects of radiation killed many early scientists. There are five types of ionising radiation used in medicine, of which the first three now described, alpha and beta particles and neutrons, are perhaps best thought of as the fragments of atoms given off by the disintegration of matter. Alpha and beta particles are produced by the transformation of matter from an unstable to a stable form. This is the process of radioactive decay.

Alpha particles

These have very low penetrating power and can be stopped by only a few centimetres of air or a sheet of paper. Since this type of radiation has poor penetrating powers it is rarely used in medical treatment.

Beta particles

These have greater penetrating power than alpha particles; they are often used in the treatment of tumours.

Neutrons

An atom is made up of tiny particles consisting of a nucleus containing protons which are charged with positive electricity and neutrons which carry no charge. Electrons which are charged with negative electricity rotate around the nucleus performing millions of revolutions in a second. Neutrons are produced not by radioactive decay but by using a special machine called a cyclotron, which disintegrates the nuclei of atoms with the result that the neutrons are freed.

Neutrons are used in the treatment of cancer and other fatal diseases. One of the advantages of neutron therapy is that even if a malignant cell is only partially damaged it never recovers and eventually dies. There are three cyclotrons operating in the UK.

The other two kinds of ionising radiation, gamma rays and X-rays, are not fragments of atoms but types of electromagnetic waves of energy; they have higher frequencies than any of the types of electromagnetic waves described under ionising radiation.

Gamma radiation

This is given off during the process of radioactive decay, which also produces alpha and beta particles. However, gamma radiation has a *much* greater penetrating power than either alpha or beta particles and can travel right through the body. It is used in a variety of diagnostic procedures.

X-rays

X-rays are produced not by radioactive delay but by special machinery. Although they are less penetrating than gamma rays they can still go right through the body. X-rays are used as a diagnostic tool to show the outline of the bone, teeth and other parts of the body which contain calcium. More sophisticated techniques exist to examine those parts of the body transparent to X-rays.

Biological effects of exposure

The human body is made up of cells, many of which are able to reproduce themselves. It has been known for many years that exposure to ionising radiation, by breaking the bonds between the very atoms of which the cells are constructed, can damage cells, that high doses can kill them, and that low doses either stop cells reproducing or damage the genetic material in the cells, causing abnormal reproduction. The effects of low-dose exposure are reddening of the skin, loss of bone marrow cells, and temporary or permanent loss of fertility accompanied by symptoms ranging from mild nausea to vomiting, diarrhoea and, in a few cases, collapse followed by death. Most of these effects appear within hours, days or weeks of the exposure, but some effects like cataracts manifest themselves after a number of years.

However, the more serious effects, cancer and genetic damage, are long-term. Exposure to low doses of radiation over a long period has two effects. First, it interferes with the ability of cells to divide, causing abnormal cell reproduction; such effects are in fact cancer. Second, it can damage individual genes, or change the number of chromosomes or their structure in a cell, which can lead to an increase in the number of stillbirths and malformations.

Dose limits

Exposure to radiation is commonly measured in rems, the present maximum permissible dose limits for a calendar year being:

whole-body exposure	5 rem
testicles, ovaries and red bone-marrow	5 rem
skin, thyroid, bone	30 rem
hands, forearms, feet, ankles	75 rem
all other organs	15 rem
pregnant women — total exposure	1 rem

It is very important to understand, however, that there is **no** safe level of exposure to ionising radiation at which scientists can be certain no damage whatever is done to the body. Exposure to any dose, however, small, carries with it a clear risk of cancer. So **every effort must be made to limit exposure**. Ideally, occupational exposure should not increase beyond 'natural background' radiation which is composed of cosmic rays from outer space, external radiation from terrestrial sources like rocks and, finally, radioactivity found in food and water. In Britain the average annual effective dose-equivalent of this kind is about 80 millirems.

Monitoring

Everyone working with ionising radiation should have their exposure monitored to make sure that they do not receive a dose in excess of the specified limits. Usually this is done with a dosemeter which records an individual's total exposure to radiation. The standard type of dosemeter uses a material which, when heated, emits light in proportion to the amount of radiation absorbed by it during exposure. In its guide, *Individual Monitoring of Persons Exposed to Sources of Radiation*, the National Radiation Protection Board (NRPB) says:

Each dosemeter is issued sealed in a plastic wrapper and labelled with the worker's name, last day of use and, if required, his place of work or other supporting identification. The dosemeter has to be inserted in a plastic holder by the wearer and should be worn between stipulated dates.

The results of the exposure should be kept by the employer and made available to the individual worker for inspection. When an individual leaves a department to work in another hospital, their dose record should be transferred to their new workplace. However, employers have to follow these procedures only where the radiation dose is likely to exceed 1.5 rem in a calendar year or when they are required to do so by the Chief Inspector of Factories. Notwithstanding this, we believe a dosemeter should be worn wherever there is a risk of exposure to radiation, and a proper record kept.

Generally, dosemeters are worn for a period of 4 weeks, although 2-week periods are occasionally used. The NRPB suggest that 12 weeks should be the maximum period, and that as a guide periods of 8 weeks or longer are acceptable only where doses do not exceed 0.03 rem in a week and that their overall exposure in a year never exceeds 1.5 rem.

Other types of dosemeter in use include film-body and neutron dosemeters. The film-body dosemeter has a radiation monitoring film which records any exposure to radiation. It has a maximum period of use of 4 weeks. A neutron dosemeter incorporates a nuclear emulsion film which detects any exposure to neutrons, and, like the film-body dosemeter, can be used only for periods up to 4 weeks.

Dosemeter limitations.   A dosemeter cannot give an instant reading of radiation levels; it has to be processed by a laboratory. But there are many situations which require an instant measurement, for instance to check that an isotope has been safely put in its holder. Normally, a Geiger counter or ion-chamber is used for this purpose.

Controlling exposure

Since exposure to *all* levels of ionising radiation is dangerous and carries with it a risk of cancer, exposure must be kept to well below the 5 rem standard.

X-ray department.   For those working here it is necessary to ensure:

• proper shielding of all areas;

- that protective clothing is given if shielding is not satisfactory (though this should be done only when everything else has failed);
- that an approved dosemeter is worn at all times and monitored;
- that equipment and shielding are regularly maintained by

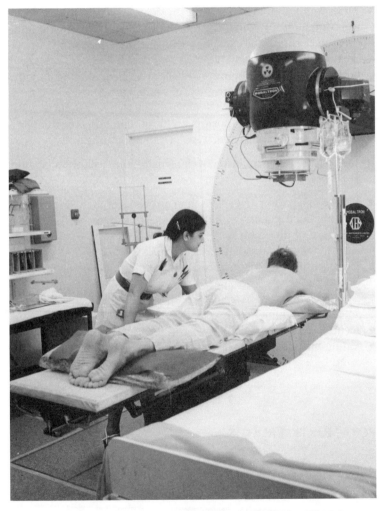

Treating a patient in radiotherapy (photo: A. Nicola).

qualified staff and that an inspection and maintenance record card is kept.

Radiotherapy and nuclear-medicine departments. For those here who handle radioactive isotopes, the following precautions should be observed:

- Time: minimise exposure time by removing the isotope from the container only when the patient is ready for treatment and, of course, rotate staff working with the patients.
- Distance: doses of radiation received depend upon the distance between the nurse administering the treatment and the patient. Therefore, try to maximise the distance between the radiation source and staff.
- Shielding: to keep exposure to a minimum, use shielding designed for the particular type of radiation in use.

If the isotope is administered internally the following should occur:

- joint consultation over handling procedures like disposal of contaminated materials, biological waste and so on;
- provision of dosemeters;
- clear labelling and isolation of isotopes;
- identification of patients receiving treatment, including notification of the type of isotope;
- employment of staff trained in the use and interpretation of detection equipment;
- accurate recording of the type and location of all isotopes;
- setting-up and rehearsal of procedures to be followed in the event of a spillage or fire.

POST-MORTEM ROOMS

All too often, post-mortem room facilities are totally inadequate, exposing staff to unnecessary risks. There are many instances of inspectors serving improvement notices on hospitals because of their poor state. One case involved a post-mortem room far too small for the workload, with poor ventilation, floors and walls cracked, sinks not provided with wrist levers or foot pedals, and no changing facilities for staff. Even the office needed redecorating. Perhaps an extreme example, but many post-mortem rooms fall short of the required standards. On top of all these things staff face risks from handling bodies, tissue and organs. As well as being responsible for the cleaning and sterilising of post-mortem rooms and equipment, staff are asked to remove organs for pathologists.

Common Risks and their Controls

Infections

Clearly, handling body organs and tissues can lead to infections. Advice on infection control is given in the Code of Practice for the Prevention of Infection in Clinical Laboratories and Post-Mortem Rooms, more commonly known as the Howie Code. In particular it says:

> When an organ is roughly handled, squeezed or sprayed with water an invisible spray (aerosol) is created which may contain an infective agent.

1. High-pressure sprays must not be used.
2. Organs must be removed as gently as possible and sectioned with care.
3. All saws produce aerosols and must be used with care. Band saws must have an extract hood attachment. Staff using mechanical saws should wear visors.
4. Ragged bone edges must be looked for and covered, for example with a towel.
5. If eyes or skin are splashed they must be washed immediately in running water.
6. All spillages must be cleaned up immediately.
7. All swabs, disposable items and material from dissection or cleaned from sink galleys must be placed in a plastic bag and incinerated daily.

As to protective clothing in the post-mortem room, the Code states:

> Clean gowns, waterproof aprons, rubber·gloves and water-proof boots must be worn by pathologists and attendants when performing a post-mortem examination.

Of course, the threat of infectious diseases like viral hepatitis is always present, so every post-mortem should be done as if a dangerous infection is present. Now the precautions which should be taken very much depend on the nature of the infection; these are set out in section 30, paragraphs (h) to (k), of the Howie Code. Guidance is also given on how to handle a body where death is thought to be due to a dangerous infection, section 30 paragraph (f). And remember, a body with an infectious disease should be kept in a body bag.

As a matter of course, all staff must undergo a test for tuberculosis as well as an X-ray. In addition, they should check to see that their tetanus immunisation is up to date. As a further precaution, all staff should carry a card indicating that they are exposed to infectious diseases. If they are taken ill the card should be given to the doctor treating them.

Knives and instruments

Again, the Code deals with the problems of cuts and puncture wounds caused by scalpels, hypodermic needles and so on:

> Cuts or wounds and needle pricks suffered by staff must be washed well in running water, encouraged to bleed freely and treated with a fresh solution of an appropriate germicide. More serious injuries may require attention at the accident department and a booster dose of tetanus toxoid. All injuries must be reported and recorded in the accident book. Any infection, however minor, following a cut or abrasion must be reported to a doctor.

To prevent these injuries happening, adopt a safe cleaning procedure. Always wear rubber clothing when doing pathology work.

Further hazards

Lifting. Back injuries may occur when lifting bodies from stretchers to tables. See under 'Backpain' in Chapter 6.

Radiation. See section on radiology in this chapter.

Stress. Occasionally, working with bodies may give rise to stress; see Chapter 6.

Chemicals. Before handling any chemicals such as formol-saline insist on instruction and training in their safe use.

Risks to undertakers. When the undertakers arrive to collect a body they should be told about any infectious disease suffered by the deceased person.

Sterilising. Every post-mortem room needs its own autoclave equipment for sterilising instruments.

Ventilation. Since aerosols are frequently created when handling bodies, adequate ventilation is essential. The Howie Code recommends about ten air changes per hour, and the air flow must not be directed towards the operator's face.

Cleanliness. Although it seems obvious, all post-mortem rooms must be kept clean. Sterilise or disinfect all equipment and clothing after use, and never leave any of it lying around. See that the traps under post-mortem tables are regularly cleaned out. Usually maintenance staff do this, so make sure they have been given appropriate protective clothing. All staff should take a shower on completion of their work.

Working in the post-mortem room is extremely hazardous; further and more detailed information on the precautions to take are given in the 'Code of Practice for the Prevention of Infection in Clinical Laboratories and Post-Mortem Rooms', available from any of HMSO. And information on the design of post-mortem rooms is available in DHSS Building Note No.20.

Formaldehyde

Where it is found

Formaldehyde, sometimes known as formalin, is frequently used in post-mortem rooms for preserving human tissue and organs. But it is also used in pathology laboratories, pharmacy departments, operating suites and renal units.

How to recognise it

A colourless, occasionally milky solution with a pungent odour, formaldehyde is highly flammable and its vapour is explosive.

Exposure symptoms

After a few minutes in a heavily polluted atmosphere an individual experiences watering of the eyes, coughing, breathing difficulties, dizziness, nausea and nose bleeds. At lower concentrations most of these symptoms are absent. Some individuals contract dermatitis as well as eczema, a flaking and itching skin. In fact, in one study, researchers found six out of thirteen nurses in a haemodialysis unit suffering from allergic dermatitis after using a 2 per cent solution of formaldehyde.

Cancer risk?

Studies with rats exposed to high concentrations (15 p.p.m.) have shown an increase in the incidence of nasal cancers. No statistically significant similar effects have been seen in other animals or at lower concentrations of formaldehyde. And no cases of cancer have been reported in people. However, a number of epidemiological studies are being done to investigate this risk. But risks are not worth taking, so try to find substitute chemicals. Where this is impossible insist on adequate extraction and ventilation systems.

Safety limits

According to current regulations the threshold limit value (TLV) is 2 p.p.m. for an 8-hour time-weighted average (TWA). This is supposed to be a safe limit but in the United States the standard is 1 p.p.m. for a maximum of 30 minutes. Of course, this points to the fact that scientists do not really know what is a safe level.

Precautions

Where there is no alternative to formaldehyde, keep concentrations to below 1 p.p.m. Handle bottles of formaldehyde with care and make sure they are clearly and correctly labelled. If a spillage occurs, remove all ignition sources and ventilate the room, using sand to mop up the formaldehyde. But for large spillages use protective clothing and breathing apparatus.

OFFICES

Although offices are safer places than factories, in 1977 13 people died in office accidents in the United Kingdom, according to HSE statistics published in 1978. These statistics confirm that offices are not safe places (table 2.1). Falls account for nearly half of these accidents while around a quarter involve handling goods. Up till now very little has been said or written about the risks to office workers, yet lack of space, poor lighting, inadequate ventilation, noisy machinery and duplicating chemicals can all combine to make the office an unpleasant and hazardous place to work. In this section we outline some of the hazards but for a more detailed account of them we suggest reading Marianne Craig's *Office*

Table 2.1
Office accident statistics

	1973–5	1976	1977
Fatal accidents	5	7	13
Reported accidents	5,062	5,359	4,926

Workers' Survival Handbook. It is important to keep in mind also that clerical staff in hospitals work in a variety of places where they can be exposed to hazards specific to that work area.

Common Risks and their Controls

Floors, aisles and passageways.   As we have just pointed out, falls account for most office accidents, causing bruises, cuts, sprains and, occasionally, fractures. These can be prevented if management use non-slip floor polish, see that telephone wires and electric cables do not cross aisles unless securely anchored, and make sure that aisles and passageways are sufficiently wide to allow free movement.

Filing cabinets.   Tipping over is the problem here, so the solution is to see that the paperwork is evenly distributed in each drawer and that only one drawer is opened at a time. It is best to close all drawers immediately after use.

Seating.   Badly designed seats can lead to backache, muscle cramp and various conditions affecting the blood circulation. Seats should be adjustable to minimise pressure on the thighs and fitted with an adjustable back rest to support the back. An adjustable footrest should be available.

Lighting.   Poor lighting can lead to accidents and eye strain, so make certain all work areas are adequately lit. In particular, see that windows are regularly cleaned and free from all obstructions. To avoid problems from glare: see that diffusers are fitted to all light sources, especially fluorescent; fit blinds to reduce glare from windows; alter the position of desks or fluorescent light strips so that they are viewed end on; remove as many reflecting surfaces as possible. If the lighting is still not good enough, ask management to have it looked at by a lighting expert. There are a number of bodies including the Electricity Council and the Illuminating Engineering Society who are qualified to give advice.

Noise in open-plan offices   This is a serious problem where there is typing, telephones continually ringing, card and paper tape punches, line printers, telexes, copiers and so on. Wherever possible noisy machinery must be isolated and placed on sound-reducing material like cork. Noise-absorbent materials should be fitted to ceilings, and carpets laid so that the office does not echo and reflect the noise. See also Chapter 5.

Duplicating and photocopying machinery.   Some kinds of photocopiers produce ozone which can cause headaches, irritate the eyes, nose and throat and lead to breathing difficulties. They should have local exhaust ventilation above them. Many of the chemicals used in some machines can cause headaches and nausea, and can irritate the skin and impair breathing; to avoid these problems see that there is adequate ventilation, protective clothing and advice on skin care, also make certain management provides adequate information on the hazards of these chemicals.

Since some of the solvents are highly flammable keep them in a metal cupboard.

Finally, training in the correct use of these machines is important, and instructions on their use should be placed adjacent to them.

Cleaning solvents for other office equipment.   See 'Duplicating and photocopying machinery' for advice on safe-handling procedures.

Visual Display Units

A visual display unit (VDU) is like a television set; an image consisting wholly or partly of letters or figures appears on a glass screen. Usually, the screen is part of a computer or word processor and is used to display information held by these machines. In the health service VDUs are likely to be introduced in the first instance as part of word processors. However, as more sophisticated medical instrumentation is developed increasing use will be made of VDUs to display information. Much of the advice given below on risks and their controls comes from broadsheets issued by the clerical workers' union APEX and by the TUC.

Common Risks and their Controls

General.   Eyestrain is the major problem, causing an inability to focus properly, seeing double or blurred edges on figures, seeing coloured fringes around objects viewed or producing an inability to look in one direction for longer than a short time. Frequently this is accompanied by a general soreness of the eyes, headaches, fatigue, nausea and various psychological reactions.

As a precaution against these problems, operators should be given eye tests before working on VDUs, and have follow-up tests on a regular basis. If your eyesight is unsuitable get your union to insist on alternative work on the same pay and service conditions. Similarly, those with bifocal glasses should avoid this work because they suffer neck and arm pains by holding their heads in a fatiguing posture. Although contact lenses can be worn, wearers training to use VDUs occasionally experience difficulties when their blink rate is reduced by staring at the screen.

Glare.   The symptoms of glare are similar to eyestrain problems and are best dealt with by the following means.

- Not placing screens against a bright window, nor facing a window. If a window cannot be baffled, the screen should be put at an angle to it to minimise reflections and contrast glare.
- Changing the position of lights to eliminate any reflections from the screen or other surfaces.
- Fitting lights with suitable diffusers.
- Lowering the brightness of any lights.
- Fixing fluorescent light fittings parallel to the side of the VDU, not parallel to the screen face.
- Using non-reflective VDU screens.

Brightness.   Again, eyestrain is the major problem which can be dealt with by fitting a contrast as well as a brightness control to the VDU.

Flicker.   As well as eyestrain, epileptic fits can be induced in some operators by the flickering or refresh rate of the screen. To control this problem, VDUs should operate with a minimum refresh rate of about 50 hertz (that is, about 50 times a second) and use what are known as medium-duration phosphors. Obviously, individuals with a known history of epilepsy should not do this type of work. Here again management must offer suitable alternative work.

Colour contrast. Although overall contrast is more important than colour contrast, yellow or green symbols on a dark-green background are the best, and cause fewest problems for individuals with partial colour blindness.

Radiation. As far as we are aware there is no evidence to suggest that emission of ionising radiation is a serious problem. But if operators are concerned then radiation film badges can be worn.

Operating periods. Continuous operation throughout the day can cause stress which shows itself up as headaches, fatigue, sore eyes and irritability. This can be overcome by regular breaks; APEX recommend about twenty minutes in every hour, the TUC about thirty minutes' break from the screen in every period of two hours continuous work.

Information overloading. Being given too much data to process often leads to fatigue in operators. They complain of weariness, depression, lassitude, anger and exhaustion. Regular breaks like those suggested above, less data to process, and job rotation where the systems need only minimal operator interaction each go some way to relieving this problem.

Layout and seating. Backache, aching neck muscles and headaches occur where attention has not been paid to the layout of the work station. To minimise discomfort, seats should be adjustable for height and angle of back support with an adjustable footrest. To avoid neck strain the distances between the screen and the eyes and between the paperwork and the eyes should be the same, about 50 cm. Also the screen and paperwork should be kept on the same level to allow the eye to move horizontally. This requires a paper holder.

VDUs and pregnant women. Reports from Australia, America and Canada suggest that the use of VDUs may carry a risk of spontaneous abortion. At first suspicion fell on radiation emitted by VDUs but tests have shown that the levels of radiation are well below the recommended standards. Since no explanation has been given to account for this phenomenon many trade unions are pressing for epidemiological studies to be carried out. Meanwhile we suggest pregnant women should be given the option of alternative work.

Although all these suggestions are perfectly reasonable it will be necessary to negotiate them with management. Plenty of evidence exists to suggest that all these proposals need to be enacted if VDUs are going to be safe to work with.

WARDS

Chapter 1 describes hospital wards which date from the First and Second World Wars, and a report from the HSE points out that most accidents in hospital happen in wards, the majority involving lacerations from scalpel blades, hypodermic needles and glass ampoules. But accidents are not the only risks to which ward staff are exposed. Always present is the danger of infectious diseases from patient contact. For instances, nurses and other female staff run the risk of contracting rubella (German measles) which, if they are pregnant, can very seriously damage the unborn child.

Although stress is frequently said to be 'the executive's disease,' it is another danger staff face. Often emotional and stressful situations occur when caring for the critically or terminally ill as well as chronically ill patients. Some patients find it hard to accept the ward routine, often verbally abusing or assaulting staff. In Chapters 6 and 7 we look in detail at the problems of stress and of assaults.

Undoubtedly, caring for the sick is both physically and emotionally demanding. It requires patience, understanding, sympathy and skill coupled with good health. Obviously, it is essential that there is a safe working environment.

Common Risks and their Controls

Falls, trips and spillages. These are a major cause of accidents. Simply by ensuring floors are dry and the use of non-slip polish most falls can be prevented. Cordon off wet floor areas during cleaning. Make certain that there are sufficient power points to stop the practice of laying cables across the floor.

Lifting patients. See Chapter 6 on backpain.

Clinical instruments. Cuts and puncture wounds are the usual consequence of the careless handling and disposal of 'sharps'. By regularly reviewing the cleaning, disposal and safe-handling procedures for scalpel blades, scissors, hypodermic needles and other sharps, most of these accidents can be avoided. Always dispose of sharps in a designated container.

Disinfectants and detergents for handwashing. Contact with detergents and disinfectants often causes dermatitis. However, by substituting less irritating substances or the use of protective clothing, such as rubber gloves with cotton liners, it can be avoided.

Stress of working in a multi-disciplinary team. Problems occur when conflicting instructions are given by superiors. For instance, a nurse can be given instructions by a doctor, ward sister or staff nurse when working on a ward, and the confusion can lead to stress. See Chapter 6 on stress.

Furniture. To prevent staff tripping, aisles and passageways should not be used as storage areas and should be sufficiently wide to allow access. Simply making sure that all doors and drawers are closed when not in use can prevent accidents.

Lighting at night. Badly lit wards often cause eye strain, stress and minor accidents. These can be readily prevented by providing sufficient torches for the night staff and giving regular breaks in properly lit rooms.

Clinical waste.   A procedure for the handling, transporting and disposal of clinical waste is given in the HSC guidance document *The Safe Disposal of Clinical Waste.*

Noise in all parts of the ward.   Noise will affect patients and create stress. Where possible, noise-absorbent materials should be used on the ceiling so that the wards do not echo and reflect noise. Regular maintenance of all equipment is essential.

Physical assault.   See Chapter 7 on assaults.

Electrical equipment.   Badly maintained equipment will give electric shocks. But these can be simply avoided by regular inspection and maintenance by qualified technicians.

Portable X-ray equipment.   See the section on radiology in this chapter.

Ward kitchens.   Often, these can be unpleasant and noisy places. A recent article (2 March 1983) in the *Guardian* newspaper describes the state of one ward kitchen: 'The ward kitchen ... is in a deplorable state of disrepair and without cataloguing the defects, it is noisy, scruffy and in urgent need of repair.'

- *Kitchen utensils.* Burns and scalds are a common cause of minor accidents in ward kitchens. To avoid them, make sure that kettles and other containers of hot liquid are not left near the edges of ovens, hotplates or worktops. In particular, the handles of saucepans should point inwards and not over the gas ring or hotplate. As a general rule always switch off *and* disconnect electric kettles before emptying or filling them. Ideally, it should be impossible to fill a plugged-in kettle from a tap.
- *Ovens and hotplates.* To prevent burns, remember not to clean them when switched on or still hot. Wear oven gloves before removing dishes from ovens or hotplates.
- *Dishwashing machines.* Removing the inspection cover and even looking inside when the machine is operating are the usual causes of accidents, so avoid doing this.

GARDENS

Many people enjoy their own garden with no ill effects, but there are certain dangers for full-time gardening workers. In particular, there are two major causes of accidents, handling pesticides, fungicides, fertilisers and other harmful chemicals in daily use, and mowing grass.

Common Risks and their Controls

Garden chemicals

Clearly, poisoning is the danger so take the following steps:

Labelling. Insist on all chemicals being properly labelled, giving details of the chemical, hazards and handling procedures. If the label has been lost or obliterated by stains, check on the contents and insist on relabelling.

Storage. Chemicals must be kept away from children so insist upon the provision of a lockable shed or cupboard to store them, and store them in containers recommended by the manufacturers. Bags of chemicals are best stored on wooden platforms raised slightly above the floor to prevent damp spoiling them. This is very important in stores with concrete floors.

Spillage.   Do not clear up spillages unless a safe-handling procedure exists.

Mixing.   Before mixing any chemicals, check that it is safe to do so. Some points to remember:

- use a measuring device; make a point of asking for one;
- do all mixing operations out of doors:
- never add water to chemicals, always add chemicals to water;

Spraying.   Use a nozzle with mesh holes 100–250 microns so that the droplets will fall to the ground rather than become airborne. If conditions are windy don't spray because there is a danger that the spray will land on the operator. As a further precaution insist on the provision of suitable protective clothing.

Handling.   Make sure information and, where necessary, training is given on possible risks and safe-handling procedures.

Mowing

Mowing is a dangerous job, especially on a bank or near water like a pond. Amputated toes and other severe foot injuries have occurred as a result of mowing accidents. Here are some of the ways of avoiding them.

Training.   If the machine is new, insist on training and make sure the operating manual is provided.

Starting off. Check for any faults before beginning a job; in particular look out for faulty controls, petrol leaks, electrical faults and loose parts. Some of the older motor mowers still have starting handles, and using the wrong grip on them may cause a broken thumb or wrist. The correct grip is to put your thumb alongside your fingers and use the fingers to turn the handle so that should the engine backfire, the handle will fly free from your hand.

Protective equipment.   Recent research has shown that noise levels linked with mowers can damage hearing. Insist on the machines being regularly serviced and find out whether the manufacturer publishes any advice on noise control. If these suggestions still don't reduce the noise levels, then wear ear protectors; see also Chapter 5.

Foot injuries are equally common among garden workers operating mowers. Although safety boots cannot prevent accidents at least they reduce the severity of any injuries. Make a point of asking for safety boots with steel toecaps.

Site conditions.   Look out for stones, bottles and other obstructions, which cause nasty accidents. Also beware of manholes hidden by long grass. Damp grass is another problem where, unless extreme care is taken, serious injuries may occur.

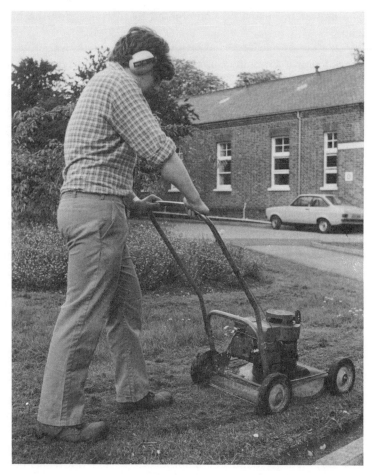

Mowing: foot injuries are common. Note safety boots (photo: A. Nicola).

Be careful when working on slopes, especially if they are steep or the grass is wet. If the mower slips away on a steep slope, let it go. In fact, it is much safer in this situation to work from the top using ropes and a rotary mower, as long as a suitable stopping device is provided at the operator's position.

If the mower becomes clogged up with grass or other garden debris don't attempt to clear it while the engine is still running.

The mower must first be immobilised by disconnecting the plug lead.

Breakdowns.   Of course, if the mower is serviced regularly, no breakdown should occur. But if one does, never repair the mower unless qualified to do so.

Cleaning.   Before the cleaning the mower at the end of the day, disconnect the lead from the spark plug so that there is no risk from it starting. Gloves should be provided when cleaning.

Plants

Although strictly speaking accidents are more likely to happen when either handling chemicals or mowing, it is still possible to injure yourself when dealing with plants. Twigs, thorns and even low branches can cause eye damage, especially in windy conditions, so insist upon the provision of general-purpose safety spectacles for protection. And if a poisonous plant is found have it removed.

Tetanus

Finally, the risk of tetanus from cuts and puncture wounds is always present; all garden workers should have a course of tetanus inoculations. Tetanus is a particularly nasty disease. It is caused by a soil germ getting into the body in wounds contaminated with soil. The wound may be tiny and unnoticed: a thorn prick is enough. The germ is also found in animal faeces, so soil which has been manured can contain tetanus germs.

On entering the body the germ produces tetanus poison which passes to the central nervous system and attacks the nerve cells. In turn this causes the muscles to contract sharply, producing convulsions and spasms. The muscles of the mouth and jaw are the first to contract, causing the tightening of the jaws which gave the name 'lockjaw' to the disease. In serious cases the onset of the disease can cause convulsions in a few minutes and lead to complete exhaustion and death unless treated. Treatment involves the use of muscle-paralysing drugs.

SAFETY CHECKLISTS

Kitchens

Is information given on the hazards and safe-handling procedures
for all cleaning agents?
Are spills cleaned up immediately?
Are all floors kept clean and dry?
Are all aisles and passageways kept clear?
Are instruction and training given on the use of all kitchen
machinery?
Is all such machinery regularly inspected and maintained?
Are warning notices placed adjacent to potentially dangerous
machinery such as slicers?
Is the lighting adequate?
Is the temperature reasonable?
Is anyone allergic to food substances?
Is personal protective clothing such as aprons and overalls pro-
vided?
Is a first-aid box available?
Are all fire extinguishers compatible with the materials being
used?

Laboratories

Is everyone informed of the hazards caused by biological and
chemical agents which they handle?
Are there safe-handling, storage and disposal procedures for all
chemicals, specimens, cultures and radioactive material?
Is there regular monitoring of the atmosphere to check that
airborne contaminants do not exceed the allowable limits?
Are any chemicals suspected carcinogenics?
Are alternative chemicals available?
Are approved containers provided for flammable liquids?
Is there a 'spill' procedure for all chemicals and other substances?
Are suitable exhaust ventilation systems installed?
Are containers provided for the disposal of glass, syringes and
needles?

Are all containers of chemicals and other substances clearly labelled?

Is personal protective equipment given, used and maintained wherever it is necessary?

Is eating, drinking and smoking prohibited in the laboratories?

Is all electrical and mechanical equipment regularly inspected and maintained for defects?

Is everyone told about the risks of the laboratory instrumentation?

Are all compressed-gas cylinders kept upright, secured and regularly checked for leaks?

Are all valve protection caps fastened on compressed-gas cylinders when not in use?

Are all manifold installations periodically inspected?

Are eyewash facilities and safety showers provided where chemicals such as acids are used?

Are antidotes, disinfectants and so on kept available in biological and pathological laboratories with instructions on how these should be used?

Are suitable respirators provided where necessary?

Are users instructed and trained in their use?

Is a first-aid box available?

Are all fire extinguishers compatible with materials being used?

Are emergency telephone numbers clearly displayed?

Operating Suites

Are all operating theatres monitored for airborne concentrations of anaesthetic gases?

Have scavenger systems been installed?

If not, is the ventilation adequate?

Is there a system for the early reporting of pregnancies?

Are alternative jobs given to pregnant staff?

Is ethylene oxide used to sterilise instruments?

Is anyone allergic to cleaning agents?

Is there a disposal procedure for all 'sharps'?

Have instruction and training been given in the use of X-ray equipment?

Are all suction lines and electrical cables anchored to prevent falls?

Is all electrical and mechanical equipment regularly inspected and maintained for defects?

Are inspections and repairs carried out by trained staff?

Laundries

Are all floors kept clean and dry?

Is anyone allergic to detergents?

Is there a safe-handling procedure for infectious linen?

Are 'sharps' left in the linen?

Is everyone given instruction and training on the use of machinery in the laundry?

Do staff have to stand for long periods?

Is the ventilation adequate?

Is the temperature reasonable?

Is there a noise problem?

Is personal protective clothing such as waterproof aprons, gloves and shoes given?

Post-mortem Rooms

Are copies of the Code of Practice for the Prevention of Infection in Clinical Laboratories and Post-Mortem Rooms (Howie Code) available?

Is the post-mortem room adequate for the workload?

Are the body storage facilities adequate?

Are the washing facilities adequate?

Is the ventilation adequate?

Is the lighting sufficient?

Are all members of staff aware of the risks to health?

Are the recommendations on equipment in section 30, paragraph (e) of the Howie Code complied with?

Have steps been taken to control infection (Howie Code, section 30, paragraph (f))?

Is smoking, drinking and eating forbidden in the work area?

Does the post-mortem room need redecorating?

Pharmacy

See laboratories checklist.

Radiology

Is everyone familiar with the hazards and safe-handling proce-
dures for infra-red, microwave and ultra-violet radiation?
Is everyone given a film badge or other dosemeter?
Are they changed within 2–4 weeks?
Are the records of exposure open to inspection?
Is personal protective clothing available whenever it is necessary?
Again, is everyone familiar with the hazards and safe-handling
procedures for ionising radiation?
Is shielding provided wherever possible?
(Note: See radiotherapy and nuclear medicine, page 42, for safe
working procedures.)

Offices

Are all electric and telephone cables covered or otherwise secured
to the floor?
Is non-slip floor polish used?
Are any filing cabinets unstable?
Is a substantial proportion of work done sitting?
If so, has each person a suitable seat?
Is the lighting adequate?
Are all windows regularly cleaned?
Is there a noise problem?
If so, has a noise survey been conducted?
Is everyone familiar with the hazards and safe handling for all
chemicals in the office?
Is there adequate ventilation around all photocopiers?
Is all equipment and material readily accessible?
Has everyone an average of 40 square feet of floor space *after*
taking into account space occupied by furniture, equipment and
other fittings?
Are all offices kept clean and tidy?

Visual display units

Are eye tests given to all operators?
Is there a glare problem?
Are there any problems with brightness?
Has the flicker rate been checked?
Is there any information overloading?
Is the layout and seating suitable?

Wards

Are all spills cleaned up immediately?
Are all electrical or other cables covered or anchored to the floor?
Has training in the lifting and handling of patients been given?
Are lifting aids available?
Is there a safe-handling procedure for sharps?
Are containers provided for the disposal of all needles and other sharps?
Does anyone complain of skin irritation?
Is ward furniture arranged in a safe manner?
Are aisles and passage ways used as storage areas?
Is the lighting adequate?
Are night staff given torches?
Is there a noise problem?
Is all electrical and mechanical equipment regularly maintained and inspected for defects?
Is the inspection done by a trained person?
Has training in the management of potentially violent patients been given?
Are all drugs and other chemicals properly labelled, stored and handled?
Is there a 'spill' procedure for all drugs and other chemicals?

Gardening

Garden chemicals

Are all chemicals clearly labelled?

Are storage facilities available for chemicals?
Is there a 'spill' procedure?
Is instruction and training given on the hazards and safe-handling procedures for all chemicals?
Has instruction and training been given on spraying techniques?

Mowing

Is instruction and training given on the use of mowers?

Plants

Are all poisonous plants removed and destroyed?

Tetanus

Has everyone been inoculated?

REFERENCES

Association of Professional, Executive and Computer Staffs (1981). *Automation and the Office Worker*. APEX, 22 Worple Road, London SW19.

Association of Scientific, Technical and Managerial Staffs (1981). Waste anaesthetic gases. *Health and Safety Monitor*, No.8, ASTMS, London.

R. Birnburn (1978). *Health Hazards of Visual Display Units*. TUC Centenary Institute of Occupational Health, London.

J.A. Bonnell (1982). *Biological Effects of Radiation and the Medical Supervision of Radiation Workers*. Central Electricity Generating Board, London.

P.M. Brown and R.V. Souter (1977). Health and safety in hospitals. *J. Soc. occup. Med.*, **27**, 148.

Canadian Union of Public Employees (1978). *The Health and Safety Hazards Faced by Canadian Public Employees*. CUPE, Ottawa.

M. Craig (1981). *Office Workers' Survival Handbook*. British Society for Social Responsibility in Science, 9 Poland Street,

Department of Health and Social Security (1974 and 1976). *Health Service Catering Manual*: vol. II, *Hygiene*; vol. V, *Safety at Work*. DHSS, London.

C. Edling (1980). Anaesthetic gases as an occupational hazard—a review. *Scand. J. environm. Health*, **6**, 85.

D. Farmer (1981). Safety in the Office. *Health and Safety at Work*, No.3, March 1981.

K. Hemminki, P. Mutanen, J. Saloniemi, M. Lniemi and H. Vainio (1982). Spontaneous abortions in hospital staff engaged in sterilising instruments with chemical agents. *B.M.J.*, **285**, 1461.

National Radiological Protection Board (1982). *Individual Monitoring of Persons Exposed to Sources of Radiation*. NRPB, Chilton, Didcot, Oxon.

No radiation hazards from VDUs—official. *New Scientist*, 27 January 1983.

The hidden danger. *Hazards Bulletin* No.17, Aug. 1979. British Society for Social Responsibility in Science, PO Box 148, Sheffield S1 1FB.

3. Ambulance Service and Community Staff

We argued in the previous chapter that instead of identifying hazards by occupation we should do it by workplace. That does not mean this approach will apply throughout the health service; there are several occupations where this method is insufficient. In this chapter we look at the problems facing ambulance staff and community nurses. Most of the hazards facing community nurses will, as it happens, also apply equally to health visitors, community midwives and community psychiatric nurses. (These staff, or their safety reps, should note that, since some of them spend part of their time in hospitals and other health service premises, it is also worth their while looking at some of the other chapters that deal with everyday problems they are likely to find.)

AMBULANCE STAFF

As they provide one of the emergency services, ambulance crews frequently find themselves working under very hazardous conditions. For instance, during the inner-city riots in 1981 ambulance crews went to the rescue of the injured, often without police protection. Helping the victims of multiple road crashes, fires and pub brawls is just part of the daily routine they face. Of course, the nature of the work often means many of the hazards are unavoidable. An ambulanceman is unlikely to leave an injured person lying under an overturned roadtanker simply because he is afraid of putting his life at risk. Rescuing people in this kind of situation is 'all part of the job'. Maybe this explains why very little safety advice is available to the ambulance service!

Common Risks and their Controls

Back pain. Back injuries are a common complaint in the ambulance service. The figures in a report on back injuries drawn up by
the HSE Inspectorate show that while ambulance staff made up
less than 2 per cent of the total health service workforce they
suffered almost 16 per cent of lifting accidents in a three-month
period in 1982. Altogether there were 199 incidents, most caused
by lifting patients in awkward situations — for instance, out of
badly damaged motor cars or when carrying heavy patients
downstairs.

Since ambulance staff are expected to lift in unusual places extra
emphasis must be put on this aspect during their basic and
proficiency training. Wherever possible, consideration should be
given to the use of lifting aids as well as safe systems of work to
minimise lifting. For example, trolley stretchers rather than ordinary stretchers are better simply because they keep lifting and
carrying to a minimum. See Chapter 6 for more detailed information on backpain and lifting.

Stress. At last, stress is being recognised as a problem for
ambulance staff, especially those on accident and emergency
vehicles. Many suffer from what has become known as 'the tension
of the bells'. Tests show that as soon as the alarm is rung the heart
rate of ambulance crews usually jumps from around 60 beats per
minute to over 150.

The possibility of physical assault, the risk of road accidents,
and dealing with serious accidents all often cause stress. But so can
understaffing, shiftwork and long working hours. All these can
add up to anger, anxiety, depression and frustration as well as
poor co-ordination and slow reaction time. See Chapter 6 for
things which can be done to relieve stress.

Assaults. All too often, patients or their friends are responsible
for assaulting ambulance crews. As a rule, never attend an
emergency call without a colleague. With mental patients, experience has shown that sufferers react best to a reasonable approach.
Kindness and sympathy will achieve more than force. See also
Chapter 7.

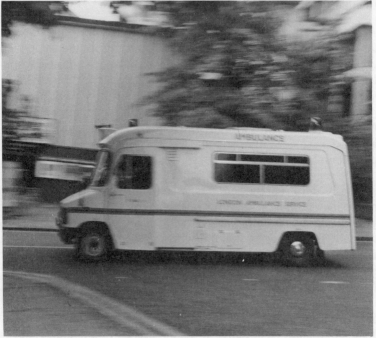

Stress: 'the tension of the bells' (photo: A. Nicola).

Assisting patients in a moving vehicle.   Movement of the vehicle can cause the attendant to slip, fall or be thrown against the walls of the vehicle. Some things which might be done to stop this happening are:

- staff training on patient care in a moving vehicle;
- joint discussions between union and management on the interior design of vehicles.

Infectious diseases.   Part of the job inevitably means coming into contact with patients suffering from infectious diseases. To reduce the likelihood of contracting a disease the following things are needed:

- Instruction and training on how to handle patients with infectious diseases.

- A procedure for disinfecting the vehicle. Check that the chemical used to disinfect the vehicle is not a risk to health. Until 1978 the London Ambulance Service (LAS) regularly used Lindane to disinfect vehicles which had carried patients suspected of suffering from an infectious disease. However, Lindane is a pesticide that kills insects like beetles and moths, and there is no evidence to suggest it is any use against infectious diseases such as smallpox or malaria. Moreover, it is a serious health hazard: scientists reckon it causes convulsions and may even cause long-term damage to the kidneys and liver. Following protests from LAS crews it was withdrawn from use.
- Medical checkups following exposure.

All staff should have a copy of the booklet *Training of Ambulance Staff — Basic Courses in Ambulance Aid: Background Notes* published by the National Staffs Council (NSC) for ambulance staff. Sections 6.4 and 6.5 deal comprehensively with the precautions to be taken when handling and transporting a patient with a suspected infectious disease.

Traffic accidents.   While attending road-accident victims ambulance crews run the risk of being injured or killed. Always wear high-visibility clothing and get police assistance to control traffic. Carry heavy-duty gloves in the vehicle for incidents involving dangerous substances.

Vehicle maintenance.   Very often, rear folding steps and cab doors are stiff; these need regular maintenance.

Control staff.   See 'Offices' in Chapter 2, and 'Stress' in Chapter 6, both of which are relevant to control staff.

COMMUNITY NURSES

By virtue of their job, community nurses work outside hospital; normally in schools, doctors' surgeries, health centres and, of course, patients' homes. With the exception of patients' homes, much of the advice given elsewhere in the book deals with the hazards community nurses are likely to face, so in this section we look at some of the problems of working in other people's homes.

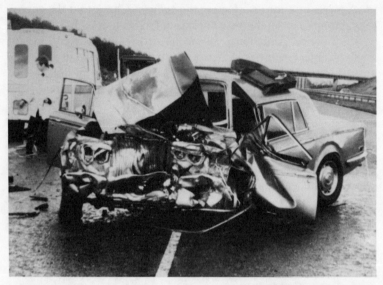

Road accidents: ambulance crews run the risk of injury or death (courtesy Press Association Ltd).

It will probably come as a surprise to learn that more people are injured in accidents at home than at work.

Common Risks and their Controls

Trips and falls. Uneven pavements, broken paths and worn steps are a frequent cause of accidents. To make matters worse, wet or icy weather makes even short journeys risky. Some of the problems are avoidable if women wear shoes with broad heels and good gripping soles. Once inside, cluttered hallways and rooms, especially if poorly lit, present potential risks. Watch out for worn, frayed carpets, loose lino, badly fitting stair-rods, small mats and rugs. Even more dangerous are wet and polished floors.

Electric shocks. Look out for cracked or broken plugs, and frayed, cracked or damaged cables on electric appliances, especially fires. Remember, faulty or damaged appliances could mean a short circuit to hospital!

Gas explosions. Gas is a convenient and popular way of cooking and heating in the home. Nevertheless, it is very dangerous so if there is a smell of gas don't use a match to trace the leak or you are likely to leave the house by an unconventional route — through the roof. Switching on an electric appliance or light is just as dangerous, as this can cause a spark that is sufficient to ignite the gas.

If there is a smell of gas or a faulty appliance, then telephone the gas emergency service. The service is free and the telephone number is in the directory or available from the operator. After telephoning, leave the house as soon as possible, taking any occupants with you.

Lifting. Back injuries are among the most common accidents for nurses. If any clients need lifting, find out whether lifting aids are available. If they are not, get help from a colleague, otherwise you will become yet another 'bad back' statistic. Don't lift by yourself. See Chapter 6 for guidelines on training.

Verbal and physical abuse. Dealing with hostile, aggressive clients, or clients' relatives or friends, is not a simple business. Try to remain calm; don't react to abusive remarks. Leave the house as soon as possible, and report the incident to management. If a client is known to be hostile, insist on a male nurse being present, especially with mentally ill clients.

Fire. Fire is an ever-present threat even in the most safety-conscious household. In the event of a fire, don't panic: just leave the house as quickly as possible, taking everyone with you. If possible try to close doors, because this can delay the spread of fire and smoke and make escape easier. Before leaving the house try to telephone the fire brigade.

Pets. Watch out for nasty, bad-tempered dogs, or other pets. Where these are a danger, leave the house and report the incident to management. Don't return until the animal is put under proper control.

Cuts, burns and scalds.   All mobile staff should carry a first-aid kit.

Unsafe vehicles.   If a motor car is provided with the job, make sure it is roadworthy before taking it out.

Clinical waste.   On occasions, community nurses need to handle, transport and dispose of clinical waste. Management should have laid down a policy for doing this. For instance, all mobile staff need 'sharps' boxes for disposal of syringe needles.

Cytotoxic Drugs

In the eyes of many, cancer is a disease of the twentieth century. It strikes fear into the hearts of most people as did smallpox and typhoid fever a hundred years or so ago. But medicine is beginning to win the battle against cancer; drug and radiation treatment holds out the prospect of survival for many who would have died in the past. In particular, the treatment of cancer by chemotherapy has meant the widespread use of cytotoxic drugs which destroy or interfere with malignant cells, without damaging normal cells. As it happens, these drugs have also been found beneficial in the treatment of non-cancer diseases like Crohn's disease and ulcerative colitis. But it has now emerged that cytotoxic drugs are a serious risk to the health of staff handling them.

What are the dangers?

To begin with, most anti-cancer drugs are known to cause cancer but the benefits to most patients outweigh the dangers. Therefore anyone handling these drugs is exposed to the risk of cancer, but this is not all. Scientists have found that they irritate the skin and eyes, as well as affecting the mucous membranes which are the soft linings of the mouth and nose.

Who is at risk?

The answer to this question is straightforward: doctors, nurses, pharmacists and ward orderlies. However, increasing use of these drugs is being made outside hospitals. Community nurses are being told to administer them to patients in their own homes.

Cytotoxic drugs

The following cytotoxic drugs are known to cause cancer and may also harm unborn children:

Actinomycin D
  (Cosmegen)

Melphalan
  (Alkeran)

Azathioprine
  (Imuran)

Methotrexate

Cisplatin
  (Neoplatin)

Mitomycin
  (Mitomycin C)

Cyclophosphamide
  (Endoxanal)

Ifosfamide

Cytarabine
  (Cytosar)

Dacarbazme
  (DTIC)

What can be done about them?

In Sweden cytotoxic drugs are thought to be so dangerous that pharmacists handle them in transparent sealed boxes to avoid contaminating the staff or surroundings. At the moment, the Occupational Safety and Health Agency in the United States recommends that pharmacists use masks, disposable gloves and horizontal laminar-flow hoods when handling them, but despite them doing this, a survey still found possible cancer-causing chemicals in their urine. So we conclude that the sealed box is the safest way for pharmacists to handle them.

For nurses and technicians the following precautions need to be observed:

1. *Training and instruction* in the use of these drugs.
2. *Good ventilation* in all work areas.
3. *Protective clothing*
   (a) Gloves: always wear p.v.c. gloves when handling

cytotoxic drugs; other types of gloves are unsuitable.

(b)   Eye protection: when preparing or injecting these drugs wear a full face visor. If this isn't possible, wear safety spectacles.

(c)   Gowns: wear long-sleeved gowns or sleeve protectors.

(d)   Masks: when reconstituting dry powder or where there is a risk of droplets being released into the air wear a face mask.

4. *Equipment*

(a)   Ampoules: keep away from the face, and when heating cover with sterile gauze.

(b)   Syringes: when expelling air from the syringe, keep the needle in the vial or ampoule to prevent droplets emerging or contamination of the skin.

(c)   Storage: store all equipment used with cytotoxic drugs separately. A special box should be provided in which needles, butterfly sets and syringes, along with used ampoules and vials, can be placed.

5. *Spills*

Before clearing up a spillage of cytotoxic solutions or powders put on p.v.c. gloves and a face mask. Then mop up all materials, putting them and any damp cloth or cotton waste used for mopping up in a bag. Seal and place in a second bag, marked DANGER, and stating contents, then seal ready for disposal.

6. *Disposal*

Normally, cytotoxic drugs can be incinerated but check that this procedure is suitable. Giving sets, absorbent towels, swabs and dressings should be put in black disposable bags, sealed and sent for incineration.

7. *Contamination*

Use large amounts of water and soap to clean any skin contaminated with cytotoxic agents and dispose of any washing materials using the procedures in paragraphs 5 and 6.

8. *Waste products*

Small quantities of these drugs are likely to be present in a patient's vomit, urine and faeces, so staff should handle and dispose of these waste products carefully.

Monitoring

Since these drugs are a serious health risk, arrangements should be made to give regular blood tests, skin examinations and health questionnaires to all staff handling them. The questionnaire should be designed to find out if anyone is losing weight or hair, or suffering skin irritations or eye infections and other complaints.

Advice

The HSE has published detailed guidance on the hazards of and safe-handling procedures for cytotoxic drugs: *Precautions for the Safe Handling of Cytotoxic Drugs*, Guidance Note, Medical Series 21, available from HMSO.

Community nurses

As already noted, community nurses frequently administer these drugs to patients in their own homes, but as stringent precautions are necessary when handling them, this practice should be discouraged. Instead they should be given only in hospital.

SAFETY CHECKLIST

Ambulance Staff

Do staff complain of backpain?
Is theoretical and practical training in lifting given?
Are lifting aids available?
Are refresher courses in lifting available?
Has training been given in the handling of patients with infectious diseases?
Is high-visibility clothing available?
Are vehicles regularly serviced?
See Chapters 6 and 7 for questions on stress and assaults.

Community Nurses

Do staff complain of back pain?
Is theoretical and practical training in lifting given?
Are lifting aids available?

Is training in the handling of difficult clients given?
Is a first-aid box provided?
Are motor cars regularly serviced?
What arrangements have been made for the handling, transporting and disposal of clinical waste?
Has training and instruction been given in the safe handling of cytotoxic drugs?

REFERENCES

Cancer treatment drugs. *Hazards Bulletin*, No.32, Oct. 1982. British Society for Social Responsibility in Science (BSSRS), PO Box 148, Sheffield S1 1FB.

John Goodland, RCN (1982). *RCN Guidelines in the Health and Safety at Work Act etc. for Nurses, Midwives and Health Visitors in the Community*. Private communication.

Health hazards to crews and patients. *Hazards Bulletin*, No.13, Oct. 1978. British Society for Social Responsibility in Science (BSSRS), PO Box 148, Sheffield S1 1FB.

National Staffs Council (1981). *Training of Ambulance Staff — Basic Courses in Ambulance Aid: Background Notes*. DHSS, London.

B. Webster (1982). *Cytotoxic Drugs and Their Handling*. Royal College of Nurses, London, Health and Safety Series No. 1.

4. Maintenance Staff

In most hospital maintenance workshops, there are lathes, milling machines, saws, grinding and drilling machines as well as a wide range of other tools normally associated with a light engineering workshop. Elsewhere in hospitals are also found steam plant, hoists and other equipment needing regular maintenance. In this chapter, since it is impossible to look at the dangers of all plant, machinery and equipment, we concentrate on most of the activities that take place in maintenance workshops, plus a few jobs done elsewhere in hospitals like welding.

PERMIT TO WORK

Put simply, a permit-to-work system is one which stops people coming along and switching on plant or machinery that someone else is in the middle of repairing or stripping down for maintenance. For example, a fitter replacing a valve on an oxygen line won't want someone turning on the supply.

Clearly, any system of work designed to stop accidents must be plain and simple, and not open to mistakes. In our example, simply leaving a notice over the switch controlling the supply is not good enough, since anyone could knock it off. The safest approach is some kind of locking device with only one key, which is kept by the person working on the machine until the job is finished, when it is given back to the hospital engineer.

If this is impossible then the following items should be included in the permit to work:

- details of isolation procedures to be given and signed by the hospital engineer;
- signatures of persons who have isolated the machinery and taken whatever other precautions are necessary;
- signatures of persons who have restored power supplies after maintenance or repair work is done;

PERMIT TO WORK CERTIFICATE

1 WORK TO BE DONE   TAG NOS.

2 FIRE PERMIT
PERMITTED AREA LIMITS

THE FOLLOWING / ARE PERMITTED	PRECAUTIONS REQUIRED	EXPLOSIMETER/O₂ TEST REQUIRED
WELDING	FIRE SCREENS	EVERY 30 MINS
BURNING	FIRE EXTINGUISHER	EVERY HOUR
NAKED FLAME	EXPLOSIMETER ALARM	EVERY 2 HOURS
POWER OPERATED EQUIPMENT	OTHER	EVERY 4 HOURS
TOOLS WHICH MAY CAUSE SPARKS		

ATMOSPHERE	1	2	3	4
TESTS	5	6	7	8

3 PHYSICAL ISOLATION
NOT REQUIRED
NOT ISOLATED AT
ISOLATED AT
OTHER PERMITS DEPENDENT ON THIS ISOLATION

4 ELECTRICAL ISOLATION
NOT REQUIRED
NOT ISOLATED
ISOLATED AT
OTHER PERMITS DEPENDENT ON THIS ISOLATION

ELECTRICAL PERMIT NEEDED   YES/NO
IF YES No.

5 HAZARDS AND PRECAUTIONS
THE FOLLOWING HAZARDS MAY BE PRESENT   DETAILS OF HAZARDS

HEAT
FLAMMABLE GAS
TOXIC GAS
CORROSIVE LIQUID
HIGH PRESSURE
STEAM
ASBESTOS
NOISE
HOT SURFACE
MOVING MACHINERY
BURIED SERVICES
OVERHEAD CRANES
CRYOGENIC LIQUIDS
ELECTRICITY
TRAFFIC (ROAD/RAIL)
FRAGILE ROOF

PERSONNEL PROTECTION REQUIRED
HEAD   HANDS
FACE   FEET
EYES   BODY
BREATHING   EARS
OTHER PRECAUTIONS

6 FACTORIES ACT CERTIFICATE
FACTORIES ACT 1961 SEC. 30/CHEMICAL WORKS REGULATIONS 1922 REG. 7 IN ACCORDANCE WITH THE ABOVE ACT/REGULATION, THIS CERTIFIES THAT:—

IS (A) ISOLATED AND SEALED FROM EVERY SOURCE OF DANGEROUS FUME, GAS OR SUBSTANCE AND IS FREE FROM DANGER; AND DOES NOT CONTAIN DANGEROUS SLUDGE DEPOSIT OR OTHER DANGEROUS MATERIAL; AND HAS BEEN VENTILATED, THE ATMOSPHERE TESTED AND FOUND FIT TO BREATHE

ANALYSIS OF ATMOSPHERE	O₂	EXPL.	ANALYST INITIALS	TIME	DATE

AND VENTILATION IS MAINTAINED, THIS CERTIFICATE EXPIRES

OR(B) ONE OR MORE OF THE ABOVE REQUIREMENTS DOES NOT COMPLY AND DANGEROUS ATMOSPHERE INSTRUCTIONS APPLY (SEC 5 INSTRUCTIONS APPLY)

7 HAND OVER/HAND BACK
HAND OVER
THIS CERTIFIES THAT I HAVE PERSONALLY INSPECTED THE WORK TO BE DONE AND THE SURROUNDING AREA AUTHORISED BY THIS CERTIFICATE

SIGNATURE	DATE	TIME	DURATION

AUTHORISED:—

PERSON RESPONSIBLE FOR WORK

THIS DOCUMENT IS VALID UNTIL   (MAXIMUM 7 DAYS)
EXCEPT FOR REGULATION 7 CHEMICAL WORKS REGULATIONS 1922

HAND BACK   Job Complete
Job not complete/Give details of Work Done

Handed back by   Status   Date   Time
I accept that the work has been done as stated and have checked other dependent Permits for completion
Accepted by   Status   Date   Time

OTHER NOTES OR RESTRICTIONS

A permit to work (courtesy Industrial Relations Service).

- signature of hospital engineer confirming that work has been done and that the machine is back in operation.

So make sure there is a permit-to-work system in operation before carrying out any work.

DANGERS OF DUST

In most workshops various jobs like grinding or sawing generate dust of one kind or another. Some materials in their unprocessed state are naturally very dusty too. The health risk is from breathing in dust particles or, in the case of some dusts, from ingesting them. It has to be said that some dusts are more dangerous than others: for example, asbestos dust kills whereas emery dust is simply a nuisance causing general discomfort. But it cannot be healthy to inhale or swallow dust particles of any kind.

Dust Control

In fact, there is no shortage of ways of controlling dust:

- It is possible to substitute less dangerous materials, for example slag wool for asbestos as an insulating material.
- Local exhaust ventilation is a common and effective way of keeping dust levels down. The object is to capture the dust as near to the source as possible. General ventilation systems in the workshop are not as effective and, in certain situations, may disturb dust, keeping it airborne and interfering with the functioning of local systems by creating side draughts.
- Dust suppression by wetting is a well-tried method. But it is not always successful, simply because some dust particles are so small that they cannot be wetted.

In addition, simple good housekeeping reduces dust if floors, ledges and machines are kept clean. Equally, dust spillages should be avoided and heaps of dust kept in bins with lids.

EYE PROTECTION

Serious eye injuries can occur when dry-grinding metal, turning cast-iron or non-ferrous metals, cutting bolts or dressing and turning metal. Usually these injuries happen because tiny pieces of metal become lodged in the eye. Unlike other injuries sustained in such processes, which usually heal without leaving any kind of permanent damage, eye injuries can cause an individual to suffer partial or permanent loss of sight. It is the seriousness of these injuries which highlights the need for eye protection.

What Can Be Done?

For thirty-five industrial processes ranging from shot blasting of buildings to electric-arc welding there are specific legal require-ments on the provision of eye protectors. All these processes come under the Protection of Eyes Regulations 1974 and apply specific-ally to work carried on in premises covered by the Factories Act 1961. However, it is worth remembering that on premises not covered by the Factories Act like hospitals the HSE inspectors still use the Regulations as a standard by which to judge whether employers are complying with their legal duties under the Health and Safety at Work Act. Put simply, if the Regulations say that a particular job requires eye protectors then the employer should provide them irrespective of where the job is done. As for maintenance workers, eye protectors are required for:

- use of hammer, chisel or punch;
- chipping of paints, slag or rust;
- use of metal cutting saws or abrasive discs;
- removal of swarf by compressed air;
- welding operations;
- dry grinding of materials held by hand.

Before choosing eye protectors consideration should first be given to eliminating or at least reducing any hazards, for instance by changing the process. If this cannot be done then eye protectors should be chosen on the basis of the type of work being done. For example, during welding operations the whole face needs protect-ing against radiation, as well as the eyes.

In fact, there are at least seven types of eye protectors, the most common is the 'General Purpose' which is suitable for drilling, light milling or up to 6-inch (152-mm) lathe work. Others are used for chemicals, dust, gas and so on.

Prescription Safety Spectacles

People with spectacles often find safety spectacles or goggles restrict their vision, mist up, cause headaches, vision problems and so on. The simplest way of dealing with these problems is to ask for prescription safety spectacles. In fact, many employers are actually willing to give spectacle wearers optically ground safety lenses, although strictly speaking they are not obliged to do so. Nevertheless, if they are provided, check that they are suitable for the job being done. At the moment, prescription safety lenses for technical reasons can only be manufactured to General Purpose Standard, and for about 60 per cent of prescriptions, to Grade II impact. This means that they are suitable only for light milling and some lathe work, and then only if properly fitted with side shields to completely enclose the eye areas.

GLASS FIBRE

Health Risks

This material, used for lagging and minor repairs, is a serious health risk. Apart from some minor irritations of the eyes, glass fibre is known to cause a number of health problems in those exposed to it, as follows.

Skin irritation. This is the most common effect experienced by workers who come into contact with glass fibres. There is a reddening and itching of the skin which is made worse in warm humid conditions. It is most likely to be experienced by workers handling glass fibres for the first time or after a break from contact. For some individuals, contact can mean dermatitis and other skin complaints.

Respiratory irritation.   Exposure to glass-fibre dust causes lung irritation, although a recent HSE report says this is a transitory effect leaving no permanent disability. But breathing in any foreign bodies must be a health risk and should be avoided.

Cancer.   Although glass fibres have not been found to cause lung cancer in people, some animal experiments suggest there is a risk from very fine fibres. For this reason alone, glass fibres must be treated with great caution.

What Can You Do About It?

Wherever there is a danger of airborne dust it has got to be kept down. The HSE working party on man-made mineral fibres proposed that dust concentrations must not exceed 5 mg m^{-3}, with a fibre count not exceeding 5 fibres ml^{-1}. But the TUC's view is that 5 fibres ml^{-1} is far too high and should be reduced to 3 fibres ml^{-1}, which is much safer.

Obviously, certain things can be done to keep dust and fibre levels down. First, find out if it is possible to replace glass fibre with a less dangerous material. Second, normal good-housekeeping practices help: the work area should be regularly cleaned and waste materials removed in such a way as not to generate excessive dust.

Although steps may have been taken to keep dust and fibres down, there is still a need to monitor levels. This should be by personal or static sampling. Do sampling on a regular basis so that concentrations do not exceed the safety levels.

Good standards of personal hygiene are also essential. For example, before washing, rinse skin under running water to remove any loose fibres. Barrier creams should be available to those who wish to use them. Finally, protective clothing is useful and can vary from simply gloves to full protection including goggles. All work clothes need washing daily, and this should be done by the employer.

GRINDING

Accidents involving grinding wheels divide into three groups; 60 per cent through direct contact, 30 per cent eye injuries and 10 per cent through wheel bursts. Of these categories the burst wheel is likely to cause the worst injuries. Most of these accidents involve portable grinding machines, and fall into six groups:

1. Selecting the wrong wheel for the job. For example, using a thin wheel for grinding can sometimes cause the edge to break away, or the wheel to fail around the flange plate. So depressed centre wheels and those straight-sided cut-off types up to 3 mm thick are best used for cutting and notching only. Similarly, grinding and facing is best done with wheels of 4.5 mm and 6.00 mm thickness.
2. Using the grinder at the wrong angle. If it is regularly used at the incorrect angle the edge is most likely to 'feather' and break up.
3. Using operating speeds well in excess of the maximum recommended speed. Clearly, grinding wheels should never be run at speeds above those for which they are supplied and marked.
4. Sometimes the guard on a grinder hinders use in awkward positions, and the operator is tempted to leave it off. But the guard is the most important part of the machine and should never be removed. In fact, it is an offence under the Abrasive Wheel Regulations for anyone to remove or alter a wheel guard.
5. As important as usage are the handling and storage of a grinder. Obviously, the grinder should not be allowed to fall on the floor otherwise it could lead to cracks in the wheel. A simple cradle should be set up so that the grinder can be left there between operations. Similarly, proper storage racks should be provided for machines not in use.
6. Finally, accidents do occur when wheels are mounted without the specially designed plates supplied with the grinder.

Now most of these accidents can be prevented by taking a few simple steps. To begin with all operators should be properly trained. Storage racks and cradles should be set up as proposed under group 5. Finally, as a precaution it is always advisable, after setting up, to run the grinder up to the desired speed. If anything is

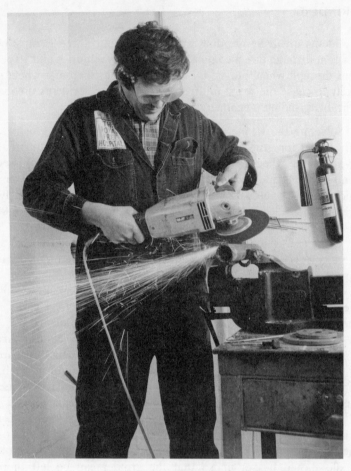

**Grinders: most accidents involve portable grinders
(photo: A. Nicola).**

going to happen it is likely to occur during this starting period.

As regards fixed grinders (grinding wheels), we advise safety reps to acquaint themselves with the extensive safety regulations, especially those covering wheel speeds, the provision of tool rests and eye shields, and expressly forbidding the fitting of abrasive wheels by non-qualified personnel.

MACHINE GUARDING

Accidents involving machinery range from entanglement of loose clothing or hair with the moving parts to the disintegration of a machine part. Clearly, these cause very serious injuries, and must be prevented at all costs. Guards are the usual way of preventing injury when all other precautions fail and, at the same time, prevent access to all the dangerous parts. Obviously, guards should not be removed simply to allow access, or to speed up the job. Further information on the legal requirements dealing with the safety and protection of workers coming into contact with the dangerous parts of machines is given in section 12–21 of the Factories Act 1961. Details of the legislation can be found in the TUC Handbook *Safety and Health at Work*.

As well as guards, operating switches should be clearly marked and easily accessible from all points of the machine. If the machine is large more than one operating switch should be provided. Similarly, it is also advisable to have cut-out switches situated in prominent positions around the workshop.

OIL

The use of mineral oil in maintenance work is widespread. Most maintenance engineers come across it as a cooling and lubricating agent for the cutting edges of tools like drill bits. The problem with mineral oils is that there are a number of serious health hazards like acne, dermatitis and skin cancer, even respiratory problems due to breathing in minute droplets of oil caused by oil mists. To make matters worse many of these mineral oils also contain additives which are a health risk in themselves.

Skin Complaints from Oil Contact

Dermatitis. This is a common problem often seen as a slight skin rash with mild itching appearing on the hands and arms. It can be more serious, and if untreated, can spread to other parts of the body.

Oil acne.   As well as dermatitis occurring, skin pores can become blocked causing oil acne. Again, if neglected, this can worsen leading to blisters and boils.

Cancer.   Long-term exposure can lead to small growths or malignant ulcers developing on otherwise normal skin. These lesions may appear on exposed parts of the head, neck, arms, also on parts of the thighs and scrotum which suffer from chafing by oil-impregnated rags. The skin of the scrotum is particularly susceptible to this, and in some instances cancer can result.

Prevention

Obviously the best safeguard is to avoid unnecessary contact with oil. This can be done by:

* installing protective devices on machines to stop contamination of skin or clothing;
* providing overalls with an adequate laundry service;
* providing washing facilities. In particular, hands must be washed before going to the toilet as well as after.

As for the risk of cancer, cutting oils are the most dangerous. The risk can be reduced by putting the oils through a process called solvent washing. Although the solvent-refined oils reduce the cancer risk, they do not eliminate it.

Oil Mists

As well as causing skin complaints, mineral oils, particularly cutting oils, can cause respiratory problems by creating an oil mist. Some research has also shown that cooling oils contain bacteria which are responsible for causing cuts and grazes to go septic and sudden outbreaks of dermatitis, sore throats and 'asthma'. The chief cause is the vaporisation of cutting oils by the high temperatures of a cutting tool on metal. This is not a major problem for maintenance engineers, nevertheless extraction equipment should be installed in the workshops. In fact, self-cleaning air filtration units are available which efficiently remove any oil mist pollution.

WELDING DANGERS

Although welding is one of the simplest means of repairing metal products, it can also be one of the most dangerous. A few of the problems are as follows:

Metal fume fever. Exposure to metal fumes such as zinc or copper oxide can cause muscle pains, shivering, headaches, chest tightness and feverishness. But after a few hours the symptoms subside.

Gases. Many of the gases evolved during welding operations are dangerous. For example, nitrogen oxide is a product of atmospheric oxygen and nitrogen brought about by the heat from an electric arc or from gas torches.

Radiation. Ultra-violet radiation is often emitted; this can cause a condition similar to sunburn. If a heat shield is incorrectly used, welders can suffer a very painful condition commonly known as 'arc eye' or 'eye flash'. It is like having grit in the eyes, and causes them to water, but seldom lasts more than 24 hours, almost always leaving without permanent damage. Similarly, the extremely bright visible light emitted during electric-arc welding means that the welder should use dark glass in his face shield.

Other dangers. Stringent precautions need to be taken when handling lead alloy steel, lead-painted plates and beryllium alloys as well as surfaces covered with amalgam. Obviously, gas welding involves the twin dangers of explosions and fire, while electric-arc welders run the risk of electrocution from faulty equipment or wiring.

Prevention

The answer to most welding problems lies in the use of good ventilation in addition to suitable protective clothing for guarding against burns and 'arc eye'. For some jobs it may be possible to use different 'rods' for reducing or changing the composition of the fumes given off during welding.

HANDTOOLS

No discussion on the problems of maintenance engineers is complete without looking at the possible risks from handtools like hammers, screwdrivers, files, spanners and so on. In their handbook *Safety and Health at Work* the TUC point out that accidents involving handtools in factories alone run to over twenty thousand a year. In fact there are some basic rules for working with handtools:

- Before beginning a job check that:
  - handles are free of splinters, rough areas or splits;
  - tool blades are rust-free, clean and sharp;
  - tool heads are rust-free, clean and sharp, and tightly secured to their handles.

- Particular points to watch out for are:
  - chipped or rounded hammer heads, and chisels with mushroom heads;
  - tools which may chip or break.

- It is bad practice to:
  - use a screwdriver as a chisel;
  - use a file as a lever;
  - lengthen the handle of a spanner for extra leverage.

- All handtools are best kept safely on racks or shelves built for the purpose. See that they are all regularly checked and repaired or replaced when necessary.

LADDERS AND STEPLADDERS

Falling off a ladder is likely to make a person almost unemployable. In fact, it has ruined many people's lives to be told they are paralysed and will never walk again. So before using a ladder it is worth spending a few minutes considering whether the job can be done more safely another way, for instance by using quick-fit scaffolding. If it cannot then check whether:

- any rungs are badly worn;
- the condition of the stiles is satisfactory.

If there are any defects return the ladder and point out the faults.

A wooden ladder should not be painted as the paint will hide defects. Instead, treat it with a wood preservative and a coat of clear varnish.

Now, most accidents involve ladders slipping. To use a ladder correctly place it on a firm, level base and set it out 1 unit from the

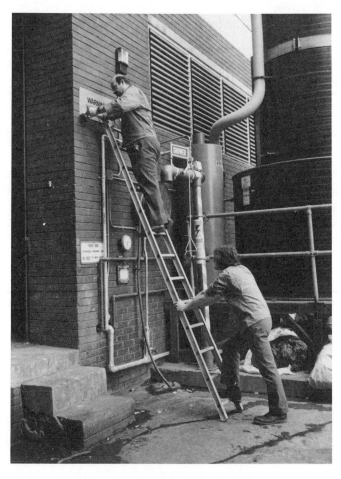

Footing a ladder (photo: A. Nicola).

wall for each 4 units of height. To prevent slipping, clamp or lash the ladder securely to an anchorage point. If this is impossible then station someone at the foot of the ladder to keep it steady.

Some of the reasons for accidents are as follows:

- Carrying tools or materials up or down the ladder by hand. Clearly, the safe procedure is to carry the tools in a toolbag slung from a strap over the shoulder. Similarly, materials can be raised or lowered by rope.
- Increasing the length of a ladder by putting it on a box or other object. Quite obviously, the answer is to get a longer ladder.

Some points worth remembering when you are working on a ladder are:

- keep one hand and both feet on it;
- never free both hands for working;
- never lean backwards, sideways or extend beyond arm's length.

For some jobs, stepladders are more convenient than ladders. Again, it is worth while doing a few simple checks before using them. Examine the condition and length of the cords, and see that they pass through the stiles and back supports and are knotted securely at each end. At the first sign of any wear or deterioration, the stepladder should be returned and the cords replaced.

Finally, when working on a stepladder see that it is spread to its fullest extent for stability and safety. Always set it at right angles to the job, that is with either the front or back of the steps facing the job. Never place the steps parallel to the job, because they are less stable in that direction.

VIBRATION DAMAGE

Like noise, vibration is a common problem for maintenance engineers, causing serious damage to the body. Most engineers come into contact with vibration problems through using vibrating tools such as portable grinders. Operators suffer from pains in their hands, arms or shoulders.

Raynauld's phenomenon, or 'white finger', is a disease which does occur naturally, but when associated with exposure to hand–arm vibration it is normally called 'occupational' or vibration white finger (VWF). The disease develops as a result of prolonged exposure to vibration in the range of 30 to 400 cycles per second. The blood vessels and nerves in the fingers are damaged and this can result in the blood supply to the fingers being temporarily or permanently impaired, giving the fingers a white appearance.

The first symptoms of the disease are a numbness or tingling in the fingers. Later, pain may be felt in the joints. The fingers will also turn white and stay like that for anything up to an hour. As well as these symptoms there is a loss of sensation and function in the fingers that will remain until the circulation returns.

Although this is unlikely to happen to maintenance engineers, it is worth noting that continuous exposure over several years will result in permanent damage to the blood vessels in the fingers. Affected fingers take on a blue colour and swell up, while extreme cases suffer ulceration and, sometimes, gangrene. Recovery from the disease depends on the length of exposure and the damage that has been done to the fingers.

The most effective way to reduce vibration is at source, ideally at the design stage. But often design changes are not possible and measures must be taken to isolate the source and prevent vibrations reaching the operator. In fact, vibration insulation or damping devices can be fitted to most tools and machines.

SAFETY CHECKLIST

Permit to work

Do any jobs require a permit-to-work system?

Dust

Is there a dust problem in the workshop?
If so, what has been done to control it?

Eye protection

Do any jobs require eye protection?
If so, are eye protectors available?

Glass fibre

Are safe-handling procedures used with glass fibre?

Grinding

Is everyone taught how to use fixed and portable grinders safely?

Machine guards

Are all machines with exposed moving parts fitted with guards?
Do the guards give adequate protection?
Are any guards in need of repair?
Are guards always in place?
Has instruction and training been given in the use of guards?

Oil

Is everyone aware of the dangers of mineral oils?
Is instruction and training given in safe-handling procedures?

Welding

Is instruction and training given on the hazards and safe-operating
  procedures?

Is suitable protective clothing given?
Is the ventilation adequate?

Handtools

Are all tools in good repair?
Are storage racks or shelves provided?

Ladders and stepladders

Is everyone taught the correct way to use a ladder and stepladder?
Are the ladder rungs worn or missing?
Are the stiles in good repair?
Has the ladder been painted?
Are the stepladder cords in good condition?
Are the cords the correct length?

Vibration

Is there a vibration problem?
If so, what has been done about it?

REFERENCES

Amalgamated Union of Engineering Workers (1981). *Danger—Your Health at Risk*. AUEW, London.
British Society for Social Responsibility in Science (1975). *Oil: a Worker's Guide to the Health Hazards and How to Fight Them*. BSSRS, 9 Poland Street, London W1.
Health and Safety Executive (1976). *Pilot Study — Working Conditions in the Medical Services*.
Health and Safety Executive (1978). *Welding*. Guidance Note, Medical Series 15.

Health and Safety Executive (1980). *Safety in the Use of Abrasive Wheels*. Health and Safety at Work Booklets No.4.

International Labour Office (1972). *Occupational Health and Safety Encyclopaedia*. ILO, London.

Trades Union Congress (1979). *Safety and Health at Work*. TUC, London.

5. Hospital Environment

TEMPERATURE

Workers in jobs where there are extremes of temperature experience a great deal of discomfort and stress. Plenty of evidence exists to show that accidents and mistakes increase rapidly with temperature rises. Most people are reasonably comfortable over the temperature range 16–24°C. But reactions to temperature very much depend on what people are doing at the time. For instance, heavy physical work is better done at low temperatures because the body generates heat whereas office work, involving little physical effort, needs higher temperatures.

Humidity is a factor which needs to be taken into consideration when deciding on a comfortable working temperature. Usually it is no problem as long as the temperature does not stray outside the comfort range. But if the humidity is too high, an individual cannot sweat properly so body temperature increases. At low humidity levels the mouth, nose and throat become very dry and it is possible to catch a cold. Indoor humidity levels should be kept between 40 and 75 per cent. Levels outside this range normally prove uncomfortable.

Heat Loss

When the body is hotter than the surroundings, heat is lost by three means: convection, radiation and sweating. We now look at each of these means of heat loss.

Convection

Normally, skin temperature is higher than that of the surrounding air, so air in direct contact with any clothing or skin becomes

95

warmer. This warm air may be blown away, or else its natural buoyancy will cause it to rise and be replaced by cooler air, in the process known as convection, which leaves a person feeling cooler. Heat loss this way is increased by ventilation.

Radiation

All bodies, including the human body, lose heat through thermal radiation. This consists of invisible rays which are part of the band of waves that includes X-rays, light waves and radio waves. For example, a household fire emits thermal radiation to the room. In normal circumstances a person loses about equal quantities of heat by convection and radiation.

Sweating

The body's most effective means of temperature control is the production and evaporation of sweat. To change a substance from liquid to vapour requires a quantity of heat. Similarly, when sweat evaporates from the skin, a quantity of heat is taken from the body. As a result the temperature of the body falls. Cooling does not occur if sweat drips off the skin; it must evaporate. Partial cooling takes place when sweat that soaks into clothing evaporates by extracting heat from the body and clothing.

Heat Disorders

On exposure to excessive heat the body attempts to maintain its normal temperature of 36.7°C (98.6°F) by losing heat, normally by sweating. In turn, this means that the body may lose excessive amounts of water and salt. This can lead to various heat disorders ranging from heat exhaustion, characterised by giddiness or fainting, to heat stroke which can be fatal.

We now look briefly at how the body reacts to hot and cold temperatures.

Heat exhaustion

This is brought on by exposure to excessive heat and is marked by fainting or giddiness. At first a person may feel tired, sick and continually sigh and yawn. Blood pressure drops rapidly, and this is followed by the onset of giddiness and, in certain situations, fainting. Guardsmen on parade during the summer are particularly prone to this form of heat disorder. It can also be caused by continually standing during hot weather in the kitchens or laundry. A person recovers quickly if removed from the heat and allowed to rest in cool surroundings with the head kept low. Of course, as we explain later, the solution is to provide better temperature control so that this does not occur.

Heat shock

When a person is suddenly exposed to high temperatures their body can lose an excessive amount of liquid or salt, particularly when they do a great deal of manual work. An excessive loss of liquid exhibits itself as an extreme thirst and fatigue, whereas the

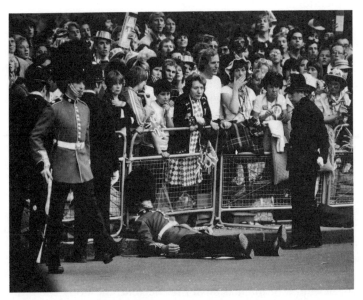

Heat exhaustion: a guardsman falls victim (courtesy Syndication International Ltd).

symptoms of salt depletion are extreme tiredness, weariness and general muscle weakness, often accompanied by nausea, vomiting and muscle cramps. Treatment involves removing the person to a cool place and providing drinks and salt to replace their losses.

Heat stroke

Industrial workers, especially in the steel and glass industries, are more likely to be affected by heat stroke than health service workers. But an unacclimatised person, that is one whose body has not adapted to the change in temperature, who does manual work during a period of hot weather, may get heat stroke. People with heart or blood diseases, the overweight and the middle-aged are most at risk. Heat stroke is recognised by a sharp rise in body temperature, inability to sweat, confusion and even convulsions, followed by a coma. Death or permanent body damage can occur. Ideally a person suffering heat stroke should be treated in hospital. But if this is not possible they should be given a cold bath, preferably filled with ice, as rapidly as possible to lower their body temperature.

Cold stress

Before considering how best to control temperature so that the environment is comfortable to work in we need to look at the dangers of exposure to cold. This is less of a health hazard than excess heat since the effects take longer to occur and can readily be prevented. In spite of this, working in cold weather is extremely uncomfortable, and ought to be avoided.

The body has developed two defences against cold exposure. First, it restricts the flow of blood to the skin, thereby reducing the loss of heat. In hot weather the layer of fat below the skin plays an unimportant role in the heat-loss process. But in cold weather conduction of heat becomes a major route of heat flow to the skin so that the layer of fat provides an insulation layer; fat people are less likely to feel the cold. Any part of the body exposed to the cold, like the hands or feet, will rapidly become numb and there will be a loss of manual dexterity. Second, the body encourages rapid muscle contraction to generate heat, commonly known as shivering.

According to scientists there is little evidence to suggest that workers can acclimatise to cold weather, although some can develop local acclimatisation. People continually exposed to cold can develop the ability to maintain blood flow in their hands so that they stay warm.

Temperature Control

Since heat can cause discomfort, heat illness and, in some cases, death, means must be found to control it. Excess heat can be dealt with in the following ways:

1. Provision of thermal insulation or shielding around machinery responsible for heat. This will, to some extent, avoid overheating of the surrounding atmosphere.

2. Provision of ventilation to reduce the temperature of the surroundings to an acceptable level. An efficient ventilation system will cause heat to flow out of the building and away from exposed workers. The intention should be to introduce incoming air at a low level with extraction fans on the roof to remove the hot air. Provision of fresh air at about 1.2 to 1.5 m (4 to 5 ft) above the ground will help to improve breathing. It is important to note that extraction fans or natural ventilation openings should be situated above the heat sources, otherwise hot air may become trapped and recirculate. Expert advice should be sought before introducing a ventilation system.

When everything else has failed the following ways can be used, but only as a last resort:

- frequent breaks taken in cool rest areas which allow time for the body to recover from the excess heat;
- provision of cold drinking water and salt tablets to replace water and salt lost by sweating.

In low temperatures the effects of cold can be overcome, and thus body temperature maintained at the necessary 37°C or so, by:

- organising work schedules to reduce the amount of time spent out in the cold;
- provision of suitable cold-weather clothing;
- frequent periods in a warm rest area so that the body can warm up after exposure to the cold.

Temperature Standards

The Chartered Institute of Building Services (CIBS) has drawn up a 'comfort scale' (table 5.1) indicating the range of temperatures (°C) over which it is reasonably comfortable to work.

In all premises where the Factories Act 1961 applies, employers are obliged to maintain a 'reasonable temperature'. Although this includes only hospital laundries and workshops among health-service buildings, nevertheless the inspectorate can use the Act as a guide to establishing whether the temperature in non-factory premises is reasonable or not. Of course, interpretation of a 'reasonable temperature' can be made by reference to table 5.1.

As well as requiring a 'reasonable temperature' to be maintained, the Offices, Shops and Railway Premises Act 1963 also requires there to be a minimum temperature of 16°C in offices one hour after the start of work. Although this temperature is far too low it provides a starting point for safety reps.

LEGIONNAIRES DISEASE

Legionnaires disease is an illness recently linked with hospitals. It was in 1976 that the disease was first recognised after it struck a convention of American war veterans in Pennsylvania, killing seventeen people. A team of medical experts from the Communicable Disease Centre in Atlanta, Georgia, was called in to identify

Table 5.1   CIBS comfort scale; temperatures in °C

Scale	1 Cold	2 Uncomfortably cool	3 Slightly cool	4 Comfortable	5 Slightly warm	6 Uncomfortably warm	7 Hot
Sedentary		14	17	21	23	25	28
Light		8	11	15	19	22	
Moderate							
Heavy	−6	0	4	8	12	16	20

the disease. After months of painstaking work a young scientist discovered the germ responsible for it.

Research is still continuing into ways of preventing outbreaks of the disease. Evidence shows that it is found in the water systems of buildings. So-called improved materials in the plumbing systems of new buildings appear to encourage the growth of the bacteria. Before 1945, plumbing networks were made mostly of iron and lead which prevented the growth of the bacteria, but modern systems now have copper plumbing that the germs thrive on.

The problem lies in devising a method for prevention. Chlorine disinfectant can stop the bacteria accumulating, so the DHSS suggest that cooling towers, humidifiers and evaporative condensers should be disinfected at least twice a year. As far as possible cold water should be kept and distributed at a temperature of below 20°C. In addition the hot tap water should be kept at 60°C and distributed at a temperature of not less than 50°C, which kills the germs. But in buildings like hospitals there is a danger of patients and staff scalding themselves. However, the problem of disinfecting shower heads and similar fittings is under study at present.

In spite of recommending these measures the DHSS are not willing to pay for them. In their circular *Legionnaires Disease and Hospital Water Systems* issued in October 1980 the DHSS say: 'No additional finance can be made available for these measures. Any additional expenditure must be contained within authorised cash limits.'

NOISE

Noise is not a new problem; for a long time it has been accepted as a normal part of the job. For many workers this is still often the case, either because they do not understand the harmful effects, or because they believe that nothing can be done about it. It has been estimated that in Britain approximately one million workers currently suffer from some degree of hearing loss due to excessive noise.

Excessive noise has been shown to cause general symptoms of stress and fatigue and to be a contributory factor to coronary heart disease and other stress-related conditions. Reducing noise would not only cut down health hazards but could also improve safety. If workers cannot communicate easily then accidents may occur through ignoring warning sounds or shouts.

But most important of all is the fact already referred to, that noise can damage hearing. Exposure to an intense noise for a short time can induce temporary hearing loss which can last from a few seconds to a few days. Quite often it is accompanied by a ringing in the ears, called tinnitus, which can become permanent. Regular exposure to excessive noise can lead to permanent hearing loss. In addition it can accelerate the normal hearing loss that individuals suffer as they grow older.

Noise Sources

Noise sources are found both inside and outside hospitals. An American survey of hospital noises conducted by the Public Health Service found that the majority of noise sources originated within the hospital. Most of the outside noise was due to the movement of traffic.

Inside the hospital noises are generated in many places. The power plant is among the noisiest of all places; boilers, fans, pumps and the combustion of fuel are responsible. But electric equipment can also be a source of both structural and air-transmitted noise. Auxiliary generators, transformers and switch-gear are the common causes.

The problem of noise is not confined to the power plant; laboratories and wards are other work areas with a variety of noise sources. Autoclaves, sterilisers, ultrasonic cleaners, dishwashing machines, ice making machines and refrigerators come to mind as common causes. Even housekeeping activities can be disturbing: witness the noise from portable vacuum cleaners, floor-washing machines and floor polishers.

What Is Noise?

All objects that vibrate make a noise. It is the vibrations which push and pull the surrounding air and, in turn, push and pull the air beyond by means of a shunting action that causes the noise to travel through the air. A small amount of energy is lost at each shunt so that a point is reached beyond the source of noise at which the energy left is so small that no sound can be heard. The waves of compressed air, set in motion by the vibrating source, travel through the air much as a movement travels along a line of stationary goods wagons when they are suddenly pushed by a locomotive. But the waves of compressed air travel outwards in all directions. These waves are similar to those made by a stone thrown into a pond. As the ripples spread out from the centre they become smaller and fade away.

Sound has two measurable properties: frequency and intensity; to appreciate how noise can damage hearing we must understand these. The speed at which an object vibrates determines that rate at which the surrounding air vibrates and hence the 'pitch' of the sound we hear when the vibrations of the air are picked up by our ears. This speed of vibration is known as the frequency of a sound. The normal human ear can hear frequencies between 20 vibrations per second, a low growl, and about 20,000 vibrations per second, a high-pitched piercing whine. Frequency is usually measured in hertz, Hz for short; 1 Hz is the same as one vibration per second, 20 Hz means twenty vibrations per second, and so on.

Most noise in the workplace is made up of a mixture of frequencies and is commonly referred to as broad-band noise. In the assessment of a potential noise level the frequency range is normally divided into octave bands, each octave representing a different frequency range. For most practical purposes the 'A-weighted' sound level is used and represents the range of frequencies or octaves to which the normal human ear is sensitive.

When our ears pick up a sound, we are aware not only of its pitch: we also hear its loudness, or intensity. While frequency is the speed of the vibration that causes the sound to reach our ears, intensity is measured in units called decibels, abbreviated to dB. It is the amount of energy delivered by the vibrating air to the ear. A scale for comparing noise levels is called a decibel scale and shows how much greater the intensity of a particular sound is than the intensity of a reference sound at the bottom of the scale. On the scale, the reference sound is set at the weakest sound a sensitive human ear can detect.

The decibel scale is based on multiples of ten. An increase in 10 dB is equivalent to multiplying the intensity or level of the sound by ten; so 80 dB is ten times more intense than 70 dB and one hundred times more intense than 60 dB. Each increase of 3 dB is equivalent to approximately doubling the noise. So 93 dB is not a small increase over 90 dB but a doubling of the noise level.

The levels of noise for some typical sounds heard at work are:

power plant	120 dB
drop hammer	110 dB
pneumatic drill	100 dB
grinder	90 dB
traffic	80 dB
loud radio	70 dB
busy office	60 dB
normal speech	50 dB

Earlier we mentioned that, for most practical purposes, the A-weighted sound level is used. This scale is commonly referred to as the A-weighted decibel scale and its units of measurement as dB(A). Most noise meters operate on this scale, which observes the same rules as the ordinary dB scale.

To sum up, a sound's frequency is the rate at which the compressed air waves vibrate and is measured in cycles per second or hertz (Hz), while its intensity is a measure of the loudness given in decibels (dB).

How Noise Affects You

The human ear is an extremely delicate and sensitive organ, parts of which control the body's sense of balance and parts of which respond to sound. It is divided into three parts, outer ear, middle ear and inner ear. Sound waves make the ear drum, in the outer ear, vibrate and transmit the vibrations to the middle ear. In turn they are conveyed through the middle ear by three tiny bones, known as the hammer, anvil and stirrup, to the inner ear. Inside the inner ear the vibrations enter the cochlea, a coiled horn-like tube filled with fluid. Pressure changes in the fluid affect tiny hairs that link up with nerve fibres which transmit electric impulses to the brain. These impulses, in the brain, are translated into sound.

Loss of hearing

As one grows older there is an inevitable loss of hearing. In most people over the age of 65 the upper limit of frequencies that the ear can detect drops from 20,000 to 10,000 Hz. This loss of hearing with ageing is known as presbyacusis. A more serious loss of hearing can occur because of exposure to loud noise. The degree of hearing loss depends on the noise level and the duration of the exposure. Two kinds of hearing loss can occur, temporary and permanent.

If the tiny hairs in the cochlea are subjected to a continuous noise above 80 dB(A) they raise their threshold of response and are no longer responsive to very soft sounds. A temporary loss of hearing happens and may last hours or days depending on the length of exposure to the noise. Recovery usually takes place fairly rapidly, a few hours after removal from the noise. But repeated exposure can lead to permanent hearing loss.

More serious is the permanent loss of hearing that occurs after exposure to loud continuous noise. When this happens some of the tiny hairs in the cochlea are permanently damaged with the result that there is a lasting hearing-loss. In this situation the ear no longer responds to the higher frequencies. Speech becomes difficult to understand because it is partly made up of high-frequency consonants like s, t and f, which are now lost to the individual.

Two other noise-damage conditions can accompany permanent hearing-loss for most workers. Tinnitus, a ringing in the ears, can be even more disturbing than the hearing loss. Sufferers find they cannot concentrate and have great difficulty sleeping. So far no cure has been found. Together with a loss of hearing some workers may suffer from recruitment, a condition where noise suddenly gets louder. Although someone with hearing loss may ask people to speak up, when they do, he may ask them not to shout, simply because the noise suddenly becomes too loud.

The social effects of hearing loss are indeed very serious, since its affects the quality of life. Television cannot be understood, music is not appreciated and speech is frequently misunderstood. Family relationships become strained and individuals are accused of shouting and not listening. Eventually sufferers become increasingly withdrawn, isolated and lonely.

Noise Standards

At the present time the standards of noise control and levels of exposure are to be found in the 1972 Code of Practice for Reducing the Exposure of Employed Persons to Noise. The Code, which is only voluntary, lays down 90 dB(A) as the maximum exposure to which a person should be exposed for an eight-hour day, or a forty-hour week. Although this is not the law it is given limited credibility by the Health and Safety at Work Act etc. 1974. Under section 2 of the Act employers have a general duty to provide plant and systems of work that are safe and not a risk to health. So it is possible to use the recommendations in the Code in conjunction with section 2 to introduce improvements into workplaces where noise levels exceed 90 dB(A).

Future Changes

The noise regulations are currently under review by the Health and Safety Executive. In their consultative document, they propose a new set of regulations governing the responsibilities of employers, workers, designers and manufacturers. They suggest a general obligation to reduce noise levels to the lowest level reasonably practicable. Workers, they say, must not be exposed to noise levels above 90 dB(A) over an eight-hour period or a peak sound pressure of 600 pascals unless ear protection is provided. (Normally, measurement of peak sound pressure only happens where very loud impulses of noise are involved, for example in industry the noise of riveting or air hammers. On instruments designed to measure peak sound pressure, 600 pascals can be taken as corresponding to 150 dB.)

More specific requirements on employers include the obligation to conduct noise surveys, provide information, instruction and training, issue ear protectors and appoint a suitably qualified person to advise on the requirements of the regulations. An employer must also produce a plan of action setting out the measures he intends to take under the regulations. Designers and manufacturers should ensure so far as is 'reasonably practicable' that new machinery does not produce harmful noise levels.

These proposals have two major drawbacks. First, 90 dB(A) is not a safe level for eight hours. Several other countries have a lower recommended maximum noise level; in Holland the level is 80 dB(A). Second, the concept of 'reasonably practicable' allows the employer the flexibility of ensuring that the cost of implementing measures to reduce the noise level below 90 dB(A) is not unreasonable in relation to those who benefit. In practice it is likely that employers will not make much effort to reduce noise levels below the legal limit on the grounds of cost.

Control Strategy

As a rule of thumb for determining whether workers have been exposed to harmful noise levels the HSE, in its booklet *Noise and the Worker*, suggests the following questions:

- Do workers have difficulty speaking to each other while working in a noisy environment?
- Have workers complained of ringing in the ears or head noises after working in noise for several hours?
- Have workers complained of a loss of hearing that has the effect of muffling speech and other sounds?
- Have they been told by their families that they are becoming deaf?
- Have workers exposed to high noise levels for short periods experienced temporary deafness severe enough for them to seek medical advice?

If the answer is yes to any of these questions, then there is probably a noise problem. The next step is to ask the employer to engage a suitably qualified person to conduct a noise survey. The results should be made available to safety reps, together with technical assistance to evaluate any proposals.

Before deciding on the most effective way to reduce noise levels, decide on an agreed standard with your employer. Where practicable the noise level should be reduced to the TUC target of 85 dB(A) over a period of eight hours. Once you have set an agreed target start by tackling the noise at source. Noisy machinery should be replaced or modified and a planned programme of regular maintenance instituted since badly kept machinery is often quite deafening.

The hospital power plant is probably the noisiest place and the least satisfactory way of dealing with this is to use ear protectors. They should be viewed as a temporary measure while steps are taken to reduce the noise level at source. Two types of ear protectors are available: ear plugs and ear muffs. If they fit well, ear plugs will reduce the noise level by about 20 dB, whereas good ear muffs cut it down by about 40 dB. The actual reduction will depend on the frequency of the noise as well as the type of protector (most items give more reduction at high frequencies). In the proposed regulations the Health and Safety Executive will be empowered to recommend suitable ear protectors, but this will only come into operation three years after the other recommendations. Meanwhile advice on the suitability of different ear protectors can be found in the Code of Practice. If ear protectors are worn, even as a short-term measure, ensure that each worker is fitted personally by a competent individual. Arrangements should be made for regular inspection, maintenance, cleaning and storage.

Finally, a short-term solution is to reduce the time of exposure by organising less hours, job rotation, rest periods and quiet times. Tea and lunch breaks should be taken well away from noisy areas. When the new regulations come into force there will be a need for increased trade union vigilance. Safety reps must ensure that employers make as much effort as possible to reduce noise levels below the 90 dB(A) limit.

FIRE SAFETY

Hospital Fires and Fire Precautions

Since 1967 there has been a rapid increase in the total number of hospital fires, as is shown by table 5.2 (taken from *Fire*, July 1981). In fact between 1967 and 1974 there was a threefold increase; however, the number of casualties remained steady. Nearly half of the fires were in patient-caring areas; kitchens came next. Smok-

Table 5.2
Fires in UK hospitals 1967–78

Year	Total	Psychiatric	Other
1967	650		
1968	684	292	392
1969	1,134		
1970	1,191	403	788
1971	1,349	517	832
1972	1,639	668	971
1973	2,044	838	1,206
1974	2,047	823	1,224
1975	2,200*		
1976	2,219	935	1,284
1977	2,148†	840	1,308
1978	1,876†	696	1,182

* Estimate.
† Totals are about 10 per cent lower than expected owing to non-reporting of fires during the fire services dispute.

ers' materials, malicious ignition and cooking appliances accounted for more than 60 per cent of fires involving casualties, rescues and escapes. More than a third of the fires involved paper, packaging, wrapping and other unspecified waste.

Cuts in health service finance have, not surprisingly, reduced the amount of money spent on fire precautions, which has increased the risk of fire. A case in point is the fire in a Surrey mental hospital in 1978. Over three hundred patients were evacuated from the hospital by the seventy hospital staff, with the assistance of a hundred police and thirty-three ambulance staff. The fire started on the ground-storey cinema stage. Fire fighting was hampered by dense smoke generated by polyurethane foam lagging to steam-heating pipes together with plastic materials used in the furnishing and for nursing purposes. Five years previously, recommendations on improving fire precautions had been made but, owing to cuts, these were never fully implemented.

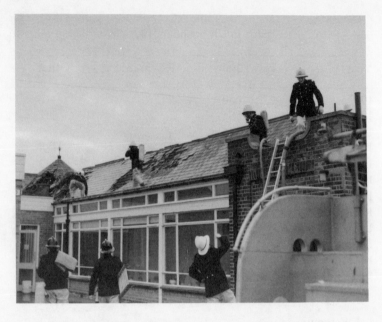

After a hospital fire (courtesy London Fire Brigade).

Unlike hotels, shops, factories and offices, hospitals are not designated under the Fire Precautions Act 1971 so do not require a fire certificate. The purpose of a fire certificate is to lay down basic requirements for fire precautions which are tailor-made for each workplace. In practice, the failure to designate hospitals has meant that less money is spent on fire precautions. According to Home Office statistics the Fire Service spent £1.3 million in 1977 on fire prevention advice to health institutions whereas enforcement costs under the Act were shown as: hotels £2.8 million, factories £5.2 million, offices £3.6 million and shops £1.7 million.

Of course, saving money on fire prevention is rash. One recent example illustrates the foolishness of penny-pinching on fire precautions. Six elderly people died in a fire at a hospital where the alarm systems were strongly criticised by fire authorities. To raise the alarm staff had to dial 666 which alerts the county fire brigade control room and sets off the hospital's fire alarms. But the fire authorities say an automatic detection system is more efficient simply because it would have detected the fire earlier.

Despite advice not to do so from the fire authorities, the DHSS decided that automatic detection systems should be used only in hospital areas unoccupied for long periods of time. The important lesson to learn here is that spending insufficient money on fire precautions can cost lives.

What Is Fire?

In simple terms, fire is a chemical reaction involving oxygen, heat and combustible material. These three things are commonly referred to as the 'fire triangle': if one is missing then fire will not occur. Before anything will burn it has to be heated to its ignition point. If a solid or liquid is heated, a vapour is given off which forms a flammable mixture with the oxygen present in the air. Fire breaks out when this mixture reaches its ignition point. The amount of heat required depends on the material; timber can be set alight only with great difficulty whereas shavings readily ignite and burn freely. So when material has been set alight it becomes a new source of ignition which heats other surrounding material, causing fire to spread over a rapidly widening area. Most firefighting practice involves cutting off the supply of air, removing combustible materials, and controlling the amount of heat generated.

How Does It Affect You?

Toxic fumes, smoke and heat are responsible for most fire deaths. In fact the majority of victims die from exposure to toxic fumes, sometimes before the fire has even reached them. Carbon monoxide and carbon dioxide are gases, present in a fire, which rapidly cause unconsciousness and death. In many modern hospitals plastics, including polyurethane foams, and other modern materials generate highly toxic gases including hydrogen cyanide, ammonia and sulphur dioxide. Of course, hospitals also handle highly toxic chemicals and gases. All fires produce smoke, the amount depending on the growth of the fire. Smoke can obscure vision, causing confusion and panic, especially among people in unfamiliar buildings like hospitals. Heat is the other major cause of death; burns, shock and heat stroke are usually responsible.

Prevention

Fire safety may be divided into two parts: first, precautions to prevent fires breaking out and, second, action taken on the outbreak of fire. All hospitals should have a programme for the prevention of fires. A plan should be drawn up to deal with all combustible solids, gases and liquids. It should cover the possibility of fire spread, storage of materials and arrangements for disposal of combustible waste. Corridors, for example, should be kept clear of combustible materials like wheelchairs, stretchers, desks and chairs. Likewise, waste paper, plastics and so on should be stored in fire-resistant containers so that any fire starting will be confined to the container. Similarly, flammable liquids like acetone, ether and alcohol should be kept in safety cans. If glass containers are required, they should be not larger than 1 litre and clearly marked.

Obviously, identifying and controlling potential ignition sources is a very important part of this programme. Ignoring arson, smoking and electrical fires are the most frequent causes of hospital fires. Complete control of smoking is quite obviously impossible. It is important, however, to control patient smoking at night, in dangerous places like laboratories and in wards where oxygen is being used. Electrical fires generally fall into two groups: those due to badly maintained equipment and those caused by incorrect use. A planned programme of regular inspection and maintenance should be instituted as well as training in the proper use of appliances.

As well as these precautions, everyone should be familiar with the action to take when a fire breaks out:

• Remove anyone from danger.

- Close all doors to stop the fire spreading. Incidentally, this also confines most of the toxic fumes and smoke.
- Use the fire alarm to alert the rest of the hospital to the outbreak of fire. In some cases it may also be necessary to ask the telephone switchboard to call the fire brigade.
- Stop unauthorised staff entering the fire area in case they hamper evacuation procedures and firefighting.
- Fight the fire. Make sure everyone has some knowledge of first-aid fire-fighting techniques. Appropriate fire-fighting equipment should be available and training given in its use. Check that everyone is familiar with the different types of fire extinguishers and how to use them. *Only fight fires if it is safe to do so*. Generally, burning wastebins, curtains, bedding and furniture can be controlled or extinguished with hand-operated fire extinguishers.

Finally, make sure that there are regular fire drills so that everyone understands the fire emergency procedures and get the local fire brigade to participate. Also, during inspections of the hospital, safety reps should ask to see the 'Emergency Service Plan'; this deals with the health authority's plans for fire prevention, firefighting and staff training for all premises under its control. Check that these plans have in fact been implemented.

CLEANING

It is obvious that some jobs are more dangerous than others but it is not all that obvious that being a domestic is risky. A glance at the accident statistics in the HSE pilot study *Working Conditions in the Medical Service* shows however that domestics and porters are second only to nurses in the number of accidents they suffer. In fact domestics face a whole number of problems like dermatitis, infectious diseases and poisoning. If you are a domestic you probably use bleach and Harpic. The chances are you had no idea that these two toilet cleaners mixed together produce the highly dangerous gas, chlorine. This is just one of the hazards a domestic faces. In this section we look more closely at the causes of these hazards and suggest simple ways of dealing with them.

Cleaning Materials

In most hospitals a wide range of cleaning materials are constantly used without anyone being aware of the potential health hazards. In fact, most of us think that cleaning materials like household bleach are perfectly safe to use. But the truth is that many of them are potentially dangerous if the appropriate precautions are not taken; for instance, when they are mixed, it is important to know what to do if some is spilt or dangerous fumes are given off.

The common complaints caused by these products include dermatitis and headaches, sore throats and a feeling of dizziness or sickness due to the fumes. Dealing with these problems usually means taking the following steps:

- Always wear rubber gloves.
- Never mix different cleaning agents together unless specific instructions are given to do so.
- Make sure rooms are well ventilated by opening doors and windows.
- With acid cleaners, it may be necessary to wear goggles and overalls. Try to find an alternative product, but be wary since it may have unknown hazards.
- Check that advice on the hazards, precautions and usage has been given.
- Find out the chemical makeup of the different cleaning agents. You need to know this to check that the precautions are adequate and to be able to give proper medical treatment in case of poisoning.

Anyone who feels drowsy or sick after using one of these products should let their safety rep know. It is very important to do this for two reasons. First, others may also be suffering the same ill effects. And second, the safety rep has to know so that action can be taken to deal with it.

Domestic Machinery

Anyone looking around a hospital on a weekday morning cannot help noticing electric appliances given to domestics for scrubbing, drying, vacuuming and polishing floors. Among the most common problems these can cause are electric shocks from faulty equipment, and back injuries from tripping over trailing leads. Some simple questions you might ask to prevent these accidents are:

- Is all machinery like polishers and scrubbers regularly inspected for defects?
- Is all this equipment regularly maintained?
- Is all broken-down machinery repaired by qualified engineers?
- Are there sufficient power points?

If the answer is Yes to all these questions then it is unlikely that there are problems.

Cleaning Procedures

In one hospital, 19 per cent of all accidents to staff were caused by falls and slips on wet or greasy floors. Quite clearly, the practice of damp mopping is dangerous if too much water is left on the floor or if buckets are left where someone can trip over! Probably the simplest way of dealing with this is to use warning signs in the cleaning area.

Cleaning procedures for laboratories

For domestics who clean laboratories where infectious material is handled there are a number of basic rules which ought to be followed. These are set out in an appendix of the Code of Practice for the Prevention of Infection in Clinical Laboratories and Post-Mortem Rooms, more generally known as the Howie Code. Since these are only model rules we suggest that management should be asked to agree the following:

- Management must provide an overall for use in the laboratory. It must be worn and always kept properly fastened. Keep it apart from outdoor clothing, not in the locker for outdoor clothing. Management must provide a peg for it in the laboratory. Take it off when leaving the laboratory to visit another part of the building.
- Do not take overalls home to wash. Management must provide suitable laundry facilities.

- Always wash your hands before leaving the laboratory. Wash your hands before using the toilet, as well as after.
- Do not eat, drink, smoke or apply cosmetics in any laboratory. Management must provide a suitable staff room for these purposes. Always wash your hands before going to the staff room for food and drink or a smoke. Never, ever place food in laboratory refrigerators.
- Do not dust or clean any work benches unless specifically asked to do so by the laboratory supervisor.
- If an accident occurs, however slight, report it at once to your safety representative and management. Details of the accident must be recorded in the Accident Book.
- Do not attempt to clear up after any accident unless the laboratory supervisor has said that it is safe to do so.
- Do not empty any laboratory discarded containers unless the laboratory supervisor has indicated that it is safe to do so.
- Do not enter any room which has the red-and-yellow 'Danger of Infection' sign on the door until the occupier says that it is safe to do so.

As well as these guidelines the following points ought to be observed when working in the wash-up room:

- Do not handle or wash any material that comes from the laboratory unless management have said that it is safe to do so.
- Do not place broken glass in plastic disposal bags. Management must provide labelled containers for it.

Laboratories are very dangerous workplaces and in the interest of safety these simple guidelines ought to be followed. Infectious diseases can result in serious disability or death.

Other procedures

Finally, other cleaning duties that involve domestics in accidents are damp and high dusting. Falls and slips are the main occupational hazards, but these can be simply overcome by making sure that when damp dusting you don't overfill the bowl with water and by not overreaching or standing on chairs and other furniture if you are high dusting.

ASBESTOS — A KILLER

As far back as 1898 asbestos was known to be a serious hazard; the Chief Factory Inspector's Annual Report spoke about the 'easily demonstrated danger to the health of workers'. Throughout the next thirty years evidence accumulated against asbestos, culminating in the Asbestos Industry Regulations of 1931. But these gave no protection to users or the general public, and precious little help to workers in the industry. By the early sixties, the manufacturers had fallen back on the theory that only blue asbestos, known as crocidolite, was the danger while white asbestos, chrysotile, was much less harmful. Of course, this has been shown to be untrue.

In 1969 a further attempt was made to control exposure by introducing new regulations covering all users of asbestos. But asbestos was back on the safety agenda in 1976; the Health and Safety Commission (HSC) set up the Advisory Committee on Asbestos headed by HSC chair Bill Simpson. After nearly three years deliberation it issued a report with forty-one recommendations, none of which has been implemented as yet. Finally, asbestos has been taken seriously by the Government after the controversy surrounding a television documentary in 1982 about the dangers, *Alice — A Fight for Life*. The programme was about Alice Jefferson, who worked in the Hebden Bridge asbestos factory for only nine months when she was seventeen, and died thirty years later from the painful, crippling asbestos disease mesothelioma, cancer of the lung lining.

Over 600,000 tons of asbestos has found its way into homes, workplaces and domestic appliances. Insulation board, floor tiles, lagging, electric insulation and sheet floor covering are among some of the products known to use it. Because of its fire-resistant properties asbestos is used in inter-city trains and on the London underground railway network. Public concern drove London Transport to remove asbestos products from its tunnels. In the health service asbestos has found widespread use in boiler rooms as lagging, and in wards, kitchens, lift shafts, air ducts and other places as fire-resistant partitions.

What Are the Effects of Exposure?

Asbestos is responsible for diseases like asbestosis as well as cancers of the lungs and stomach. The cripping disease asbestosis, where the soft lung tissue becomes scarred, is usually fatal. Often the victim suffers from other respiratory illness as well, such as TB, bronchitis and/or pneumonia, all of which may eventually prove fatal. Mesothelioma, a once-rare cancer of the stomach and lung linings, is always fatal and almost exclusively linked with exposure to asbestos. Like smoking, asbestos fibres are responsible for lung cancer.

What Are Safe Levels?

In 1969 the safe level was thought to be two asbestos fibres per millilitre of air. But this 'safe' level, based on a study of 290 Rochdale asbestos workers, was arrived at through serious statistical and measurement errors. According to this study the risk of a worker contracting asbestosis in a 'two fibre' asbestos factory was one in a hundred; in fact, correct calculations show that it is one in four or five. So the so-called safe level was incorrect, by a factor of twenty or twenty-five.

Since then the HSC has set a new lower level of one fibre per millilitre for white asbestos but some scientists reckon that even this carries a one-in-a-hundred or one-in-fifty risk of death.* In fact, if this level were halved a worker would still end up breathing in some four million fibres every working day. So the GMBATU, which represents most asbestos workers, say the level should be set at 0.2 of a fibre, one-fifth of the new level. For the general public the union suggests the level should be one-fiftieth of a fibre.

But the view of the US government agency responsible for health and safety is that 'There is no evidence for a safe level of asbestos exposure. Even at very short periods, one day to three

---

* The control limits (fibres per millilitre) are: blue asbestos, 0.2; brown, 0.5; white, 1.0. They apply when measured as a time-weighted average over any four-hour period.

months, significant disease can occur.' Plenty of evidence exists to support this view. Nancy Tait, whose husband died of mesothelioma even though his exposure was only three or four hours every four to six months, has turned up numerous cases of chance exposure that have led to asbestos-related diseases such as those of the man who spent one day building a shed from asbestos sheets, or the woman who lived in the same house as an asbestos worker. Her booklet *Asbestos Kills* describes many other cases. Alan Dalton, author of the well-researched book *Asbestos Killer Dust*, believes that any safe level is quite arbitrary. Clearly, the safest level is no exposure at all.

How Do You Identify Asbestos?

Unfortunately, there is no easy way. As a first step, approach management and ask whether asbestos has been used in the construction of any buildings. If there is any doubt, insist on a survey to identify all possible sources. Where there is any uncertainty as to whether a material is in fact asbestos, samples for analysis should be taken by management with the safety rep present. Various companies exist to do this and can give advice on removal procedures.

Remember that it is the asbestos fibres which are dangerous; they are so small that an electron microscope is required to magnify them enough so that the individual fibres can be seen. They are so tiny that one gram of asbestos fibres, laid end to end, would reach the moon and it is these which enter the lungs and kill their victims.

What Can Be Done About It?

If asbestos is discovered it can be stripped out or sealed. Obviously, the safest solution is stripping, particularly where it may be flaking or crumbling. Since this is expensive a number of 'cowboy' contractors, willing to save money by taking risks, are available to do the work. Clearly, this is not acceptable; only reputable contractors employing the precautions set out in the HSE booklet *Work with Asbestos Insulation and Asbestos Coating* should be

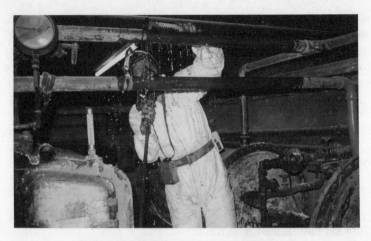

**Asbestos removal (courtesy Institute of
Occupational Medicine, Edinburgh)**

used. This publication provides practical guidance on the safe-handling procedures to be followed when stripping asbestos. Safety reps should get themselves a copy so that they know whether contractors are following the right procedures.

Instead of removing asbestos, management may prefer sealing it simply because it is cheaper. But an American survey of sealed-in asbestos, reported in *Hospital Asbestos Hazards*, by the Hospital Hazards Group of the British Society for Social Responsibility in Science, suggested that seals were easily broken. Nevertheless, where the asbestos is not subject to disturbance or vibration, sealing may be an acceptable solution. Again, the HSE booklet gives advice on the precautions to take as well as guidance on types of sealant. Wherever this is done, don't forget to have:

- all sealed panels labelled 'Asbestos Hazard';
- a permit-to-work system operating for maintenance jobs;
- regular union inspections for damage.

All the same, sealing should be seen as a short-term solution; **the aim should be the phased removal of all asbestos, irrespective of its state, from the workplace.**

SAFETY CHECKLISTS

Temperature

Is the temperature reasonable?
Is a thermometer available to measure it?
If the temperature is too high:
- Is all equipment and machinery thermally insulated?
- Is there any ventilation?
- Has expert advice been sought by management on the ventilation?
- As a last resort:
  Are regular breaks given?
  Are cold drinks and salt tablets readily available?
If the temperature is too low:
- Is cold weather clothing provided?
- Are frequent breaks in a warm rest area given?

Legionnaires Disease

Are water cooling towers, humidifiers and evaporative condensers
disinfected at least twice a year?

Noise

Is there a noise problem?
Has a noise survey been done?
Has a noise standard been agreed?
Can the noise be tackled at source?
As a last resort:
- Are ear defenders available?
- Are these fitted by a qualified person?
- Are arrangements made for them to be regularly inspected,
  maintained and cleaned?
- Are proper storage facilities available?

Fire

Prevention

Is the 'emergency service plan' available for inspection?
Are there regular fire drills involving the fire brigade?
Is there a hospital fire-prevention programme?
Are special arrangements made for flammable materials and liquids?
Is smoking kept strictly under control?
Is all electrical equipment regularly inspected and maintained?

Precautions

Are all fire exits free from obstruction and clearly marked?
Is the fire alarm audible in all parts of the hospital buildings?
Is the fire alarm regularly tested?
Are there regular fire drills?

Firefighting

Is firefighting equipment provided?
Is it suitable for the fire risks involved?
Has anyone been trained to use the equipment?

Cleaning

Is everyone told how to use cleaning agents correctly?
Are all cleaning agents properly labelled?
What instruction and training has been given in the use of domestic machinery?

Cleaning Procedures in Laboratories

Has instruction and training in cleaning procedures been given?
Is the cleaning supervised?
Are overalls available for use only in laboratories?
Are lockers for outdoor clothing available outside the laboratories?
Are pegs available inside the laboratories for overalls?

Asbestos

Has asbestos been used in the construction of hospital buildings?
If so, what arrangements have been made to deal with it?
Who is responsible for sealing or stripping any asbestos?

REFERENCES

Asbestos

Asbestos kills. *Nursing Times*, 6 May 1976
A. Dalton (1979). *Asbestos Killer Dust—A Worker/Community Guide: How to Fight the Hazards of Asbestos and Its Substitutes.* British Society for Social Responsibility in Science, 9 Poland Street, London W1
Hospital Hazards Group (1980). *Hospital Asbestos Hazards.* British Society for Social Responsibility in Science, 9 Poland Street, London W1
D. Nicholson-Lord (1982). Asbestos: a total ban could be the only answer. *The Times*, 28 August 1982
N. Pollitt (1982). Asbestos—licence to kill renewed. *New Statesman*, 27 August 1982
N. Tait (1976). *Asbestos Kills.* The Silbury Fund, 24 Rivermill, London SW1V 3JN

Cleaning

J.A. Lunn (1976). *The Health of Staff in Hospitals.* Heinemann Medical Books, London
South Western Regional Health Authority (1977). *Health and Safety at Work: A Guide to the Act for Domestic Staff in the Health Service.* SWRHA, Bristol

Fire

R.G. Bond, G.S. Michaelson and R.L. De Roos (1973). *Environmental Health and Safety in Health Care Facilities.* Collier-Macmillan, London.

S.E. Chandler (1981). Statistics brought up to date. *Fire*, July 1981
Conference on fire safety in hospitals and nursing homes. *Fire Prevention*, Dec. 1978
Death ward alarms had government approval. *Safety*, Oct. 1980
Mental hospital fire. *Fire Prevention*, No.128, 1978, p.41
'Phoenix' (nom de plume) (1981). Designation: 'Grey Book' view. *Fire*, July 1981

Noise

P. Sutton (1980). Noise and hearing. *Handbook of Occupational Hygiene*, vol.1, 2.2.2.01–2.2.2.11
R.G. Bond, G.S. Michaelson and R.L. De Roos (1973). *Environmental Health and Safety in Health Care Facilities*. Collier-Macmillan, London
Department of Employment (1974). *Noise and the Worker*. Health and Safety at Work Booklet No.25

Temperature

D.A. McIntyre (1980), *Indoor Climate*. Applied Science Publishers, London

6.   Stress and Backpain

STRESS

In the past, little attention has been paid to stress as an occupational hazard, and only managers were thought to suffer from it. Consequently the subject of stress and its effect on workers' health has been neglected. But some 37 million working days are lost every year through stress-related illnesses whereas about 23 million days are lost through accidents at work, according to Mackay and Cox in *Stress at Work*, Chapter 7. In fact mental illnesses are increasing more rapidly than those due to any other cause.

Physical health as well as mental health is affected by stress. Ample evidence is available to show that coronary heart disease is related to stress as are high blood pressure, ulcers, asthma and diabetes. Among those with a higher than average death-rate from heart disease are train guards, ambulance staff, police and maintenance fitters. Of course, stress is not always the only cause but it is a factor which can no longer be ignored.

What is Stress?

Before discussing the causes and results of stress we should attempt to define it. This is more difficult than it may appear at first since there is no single definition acceptable to everyone. Without involving ourselves in technical jargon we will consider stress to be the result of an imbalance between, on the one hand, the demands on a person and, on the other, their ability to cope with them. From this definition it is clear that many people have jobs which cause stress in which they experience, for example, pressure of work, artificial deadlines, or monotonous and/or dangerous work. Long-term exposure to stresses like these can have a serious effect on the mental and physical health of workers.

As part of everyday life, stress is not something to be avoided at all costs. The excitement of a football match or horse race sets the adrenalin flowing, but most of us would not be without them. What we are concerned about here are those factors which create stress in jobs and which can be avoided.

Although a great deal of research has been done on the causes and effects of stress among managers, few studies have dealt with health service workers. This is surprising since nurses, for instance, regularly have to deal with awkward patients unwilling to accept the hospital routine and only too willing to abuse or assault them. What little research has been done confirms the view that the most stressful situations involve staff with direct patient-care responsibilities. Nurses often feel overloaded with work, unable to influence administrative decisions or burdened with continually conflicting demands. In fact too much energy is spent dealing with these problems and not enough on the immediate task.

In one American study a high turnover of nurses was found in the newborn intensive-care unit of a hospital. Researchers found

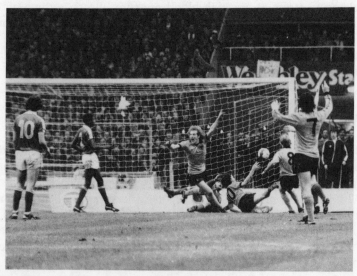

A football match sets the adrenalin flowing (courtesy Syndication International Ltd).

that the excitement and stress which attracted a nurse to this work was also the same excitement and stress which ultimately drove her/him away. Other researchers have identified two particular causes of stress affecting nurses:

- the dump-on syndrome where nurses felt that doctors were overloading them with admissions at a time when they were working to full capacity;
- overwork because they found themselves working on their days off and at weekends.

Many ambulance staff find they suffer from what has become commonly known 'tension of the bells'. While at rest a person's normal heartbeat is around 40 beats per minute, reaching between 60 and 80 for ordinary activities. However, tests on ambulance staff have shown heartbeats in the region of 150-plus at the sound of the alarm when answering emergency calls. Generally, this lasts for up to ten minutes before returning to normal. It takes about eighteen months to get used to this stress. Of course, no one knows what are the long-term effects on health. It is worth noting that their home life is also badly affected: they tend to over-react to the screeching of brakes or a ringing telephone.

In this chapter we look at some causes and effects of stress in health workers and, in turn, on the steps trade unionists can take to minimise or prevent it. We begin by examining some of the common causes of stress.

Causes of Stress at Work

In a review of stress undertaken for the Department of Employment, twenty-six factors were identified as possible causes of stress, all of which can contribute to mental ill health, physical illnesses and the disruption of a worker's family and social life. Out of these factors we focus on those which are most likely to affect health service workers, in particular low pay, overtime and shiftwork, job satisfaction, organisational structure and physical environment.

Low pay

In 1982 the average non-manual gross wage of men was £179; male nurses in the NHS earned an equivalent of £131 and female nurses £105. Ancillary workers found themselves in a similar situation: the average manual gross wage for men was £154 while for male and female ancillary workers it was £104 and £82 respectively. Overtime pay, shiftwork premiums and productivity bonuses all go to making this up. If we ignore overtime and shiftwork payments the pay of male and female nurses drops to the meagre sums of £113 and £95.50, respectively. Clearly, in comparison with the rest of the working population, NHS non-medical staff are low paid with the result that they suffer from the stresses of dependence on overtime and shiftwork premiums to provide a living wage.

Overtime

Overtime is widespread among non-medical staff in the health service. According to the New Earnings Survey for 1982 male ancillary staff worked an average of 5 hours overtime each week, increasing their average gross weekly pay by just over a sixth. A more detailed breakdown of pay in the 1981 New Earnings Survey showed that male hospital porters worked an average of 9½ hours overtime each week thereby increasing their gross weekly wage by just under a third.

Excessive overtime has several well-documented effects. Working long hours leads to chronic fatigue, a feeling of being tired throughout the day. Workers commonly experience drowsiness and an inability to concentrate, often accompanied by aches and pains, leading to a state of anxiety and depression. Less time is spent with friends and families, creating emotional stress through loneliness and isolation.

Shiftwork

For those on shiftwork, unsocial hours can affect their health, both physical and mental. In particular it disrupts sleep patterns, affects digestion, induces fatigue and varies the body's biological rhythms. Nervous disorders, particularly depression, are also common. All these combine to cause ill health and allow stress to build up.

Sleep patterns.   Shiftworkers invariably sleep less during the day than they would at night, their sleep is often disrupted by daytime activities like neighbours calling, and the quality is poorer. All these contribute to a sleep debt, a build-up of inadequate sleep over the nightwork period. Researchers have found that over half of all shiftworkers suffer from sleep disorders.

Digestion.   Some studies support the view that shiftworkers are prone to indigestion and gastric disorders, including ulcers. Irregular mealtimes and stress are probably important factors in causing these.

Fatigue.   Most shiftworkers suffer from chronic fatigue, an inability to concentrate, drowsiness and a feeling of being generally run down. Not surprisingly, more mistakes occur at night, sometimes causing serious accidents.

Biological rhythms.   Most of the body's functions — eating, sleeping and other physiological functions — follow a daily pattern known as circadian rhythms or, more commonly, biological rhythms. These cycles relate to the activities that happen about us; for example, we eat at about the same time as everyone else in the community. Shiftwork seriously disrupts these patterns, and the body adapts only slowly to the change. Rest days bring back the normal pattern of activity so that the body must again adapt on beginning work.

Nervous disorders.   Many shiftworkers suffer 'night worker's neurosis', a feeling of weakness, with insomnia frequently accompanied by irritability and depression.

Not all shiftworkers suffer ill health but most find that their family and social life is severely disrupted. If a husband or wife is on shiftwork marital relationships suffer, sometimes leading to a breakdown of the marriage. For women with the responsibility for a family, shiftwork creates particular difficulties. For instance, they have to ensure that the general running of the home is not disrupted. Of course, the social life of all shiftworkers is affected since most leisure activities fit in with the normal working week. Persons living alone are most vulnerable to social isolation and should think carefully about accepting shiftwork.

Job satisfaction

Nowadays we hear a great deal about job satisfaction without very much being done to improve it for most workers. A failure to get satisfaction can readily contribute to an experience of stress. A feeling of dissatisfaction can lead to ill health as well as high absenteeism, industrial disputes and accidents, so it is important to find out what makes a job satisfying to an individual. Among the factors most likely to determine whether an individual has job satisfaction are the following.

A challenging job. Problems can arise unless a job is mentally challenging and within a person's capability. A job that is monotonous and repetitive is most likely to create stress. Without a challenge the possibility of an individual using their intelligence and creativity is removed; this creates frustration and boredom leading to stress. Of course, a person must be able to cope successfully with his work otherwise he will find himself under pressure and stress very quickly builds up.

Interest in the job. A job that is monotonous and routine readily creates a state of stress. A person must find some interest in their work if they are to avoid a feeling of frustration and tension. For most workers this is obviously difficult simply because the nature of the job is dull and repetitive. But involvement in decisions on how the job is to be done can create a sense of fulfillment.

Pay. Unless pay reflects the skill and responsibilities that are expected of an individual, disillusionment may set in to the point where problems arise. Earlier in this chapter we dealt with the problem of low pay.

Working conditions. A monotonous job is made much worse if the working conditions are unsatisfactory. If it is too noisy to chat or too cold to work the job becomes intolerable. Instead, the working conditions must be such as to allow the job to be done satisfactorily without any discomfort. See the section below on physical environment for more details.

Self-esteem. An individual must feel that his/her job is important and making a positive contribution to the running of the organisation. Everyone must feel that they have a part to play, otherwise they will quickly lose interest in their work, which can often create stress.

If some or all of these factors are not met an individual is likely to be dissatisfied with his/her job.

Organisational structure

Like other industries the health service has a hierarchical work structure; the work of the organisation is divided into individual jobs that slot into a pyramid structure. Except at the top and bottom of the pyramid each worker is responsible to the level above and, at the same time, controls the level below. A ward sister, for example, controls and organises the work of the nurses in her ward but is, in turn, responsible to a nursing officer. Similarly, a chef is responsible for hospital kitchen staff and is accountable to the catering manager. Of course, this is an over-simplification of a complex bureaucratic hierarchy but it allows us to examine some of the ways in which tension, strain and conflict occur. The main reasons are the following:

- Role conflict: may occur if conflicting instructions are given by superiors or tasks are outside an individual's job description.
- Role ambiguity: may arise where the work objectives are unclear, where the worker is not aware of what colleagues' and superiors' expectations are, or where they do not understand the requirements and responsibilities of the job.
- Responsibility: too much can lead to serious ill health.
- Conflicts with superiors.
- In the health service it is possible to be continually crossing organisational divisions. Porters, for example, assisting in a ward, are responsible to the head porter and to the ward sister.

Physical environment

Heat, noise and lighting are among the range of stress-related factors that affect the body.

Heat. More accidents and mistakes occur in uncomfortable temperatures, especially heat. They occur as a result of irritability, fatigue, awkwardness and stress. In hot weather the body reacts differently to heat. Response is governed by the level of activity, conditions of exposure and individual reactions. At one end of the scale a person may suffer heat exhaustion, which generally shows itself as lassitude, irritability and fatigue. The other extreme is characterised by heat stroke where there is a sharp rise in the body temperature, delirium, confusion and, occasionally convulsions. Consult Chapter 5 for further details.

Noise. A Swedish study has shown that workers exposed to loud noise suffer from higher rates of hypertension. Other researchers have found that workers in noisy workplaces suffer more emotional tension, both at home and at work. As well as inducing stress, loud noise is annoying, prevents conversation and damages hearing. Further details on the hazards involved are given in Chapter 5.

Lighting. Poor lighting can also increase stress as well as causing eye strain, fatigue and headaches. Glare is another factor which can cause stress.

Stress and ill Health

There is little doubt that stress is responsible for a wide range of illnesses. Headaches, insomnia and indigestion are often the early symptoms. If the stress goes on for long periods the effects are more harmful.

Hypertension. In stressful situations there is often an increase in blood pressure due to a narrowing of the blood vessels. Usually, when the causes of stress are removed the blood pressure returns to normal. Where stress remains for long periods as, for example, in casualty, blood pressure remains high. This condition is known as hypertension and is a contributory factor to heart disease.

Coronary heart disease.   Strain and pressure can also lead to this by increasing the amount of fatty acids in the blood stream. In the absence of physical activity this can be converted to deposits of fat and cholesterol on the walls of the arteries, causing a narrowing and clogging. When this happens a blockage of the arteries is more likely to occur, leading to a heart attack.

Bronchial asthma.   More controversial is the view that stress is a factor in asthma. Some researchers have found that asthma attacks can be brought on by exposure to emotional stress, although many doctors discount this.

Diabetes.   Research has shown that diabetes lies dormant in some people and that exposure to stress can bring the symptoms on. If, however, stress were the only factor then many more people would develop the disease. It is interesting to note that diabetics can on the whole cope with stress better than non-diabetics.

Ulcers.   Peptic ulcers often occur as a result of stress. Although the mechanism is not clearly understood, stress is said to reduce the resistance of the intestinal lining to gastric-acid secretion from the stomach. This may lead to ulcers in the upper part of the intestinal tract.

The psychological well being of those under stress for long periods can be affected. In general the following symptoms are seen:

Anxiety.   Anxiety may arise through working with the terminally ill, working in intensive-care units or dealing with awkward and violent patients. Of course, anxiety is a normal response to crises but there is a point when it becomes unbearable and something has to be done. Too much anxiety leads to an inability to concentrate, depression, a tendency to be sensitive to criticism and, in some cases, hysteria. An anxious person often suffers from poor sleep and nightmares as well as tenseness and sweating. Quite often these feelings affect their family and social life.

Fatigue.   Tiredness from overwork and the emotional responsibilities of caring for the sick cause fatigue. Workers suffering from exhaustion commonly experience an inability to concentrate plus a feeling of drowsiness, often accompanied by aches and pains.

Depression. Many people suffer from bouts of mild depression but, under normal circumstances, they recover quite quickly. Sometimes, of course, the depression does not lift. This is particularly true if it comes about as a result of chronic fatigue and anxiety. Here a feeling of failure and hopelessness can go on for months. The depressed person has difficulty in getting off to sleep and wakes early in the morning. A loss of appetite and a feeling of lethargy and listlessness following poor sleep are quite common. In some cases the depressed person may be slow in thinking and taking decisions.

Aggression. Stress can affect working relationships. When a worker feels that a situation is becoming increasingly difficult to cope with, resentment builds up. An outburst of violent feelings can be the result of such accumulated tensions, and is often directed towards those not responsible.

Drug abuse. Some people faced with stressful situations at work turn to drugs to help them cope. They may use socially acceptable drugs like alcohol and tobacco or tranquillisers and antidepressants given by their doctor. A few people may even turn to illegal drugs such as cannabis. Although they may relieve the symptoms of strain, drugs do not remove the underlying causes. There is also the danger that drugs like alcohol or cannabis can affect an individual's ability to do their job as well as opening the door to physical and psychological dependence.

How Stress Affects Health Service Workers

Most jobs in the health services have some of the factors identified as causes of stress; low pay, involuntary overtime and shiftwork are obvious examples. For ancillary workers like hospital porters, kitchen assistants and laundry staff there is very little job satisfaction; the work is invariably monotonous and routine. Also ancillary workers are not made to feel that their jobs are important to the running of the hospital.

For nurses there is the problem of coping with the sick every day. Too much pressure of this kind can create stress. The pay nurses receive does not in any way reflect the skills and responsibilities expected of them, and although they know that their work is essential, nurses are not encouraged to feel an important part of the health-care team.

Ambulance crews also face problems which bring great pressure on them. At the beginning of this chapter we mentioned the syndrome of the 'tension of the bells' which is a problem other health service staff do not have to face. Their work involves long periods of relative inactivity punctuated by short periods of intense physical and mental effort at the scenes of accidents and other tragedies which gives rise to stress.

The hierarchical structure of the health services can, as we have said earlier, lead to difficulties of role conflict, role ambiguity and the problems of crossing organisational divisions. These situations can be sources of conflict, creating feelings of anxiety and frustration.

All of these factors acting independently or together can cause any of the stress-related illnesses described in the previous section. In turn, this can lead to strains within the family as well as a gradual isolation from friends and relatives.

What Can Be Done?

In this chapter we have identified the main causes of stress; now we look at some of the ways in which they can be dealt with. Low pay and the associated problems of overtime and shiftwork are not easy to solve. In private industry these could be readily dealt with using the collective bargaining strength of the trade unions. However, in the health service effective industrial action is likely to harm patients, so there is a reluctance on the part of health service workers to embark on this course of action.

A twofold strategy involving support of the wider trade union movement, and a recognition by government that there should be some basic level of pay which no one should fall below, has most chance of success. For many years NUPE has argued for a minimum wage of two-thirds average earnings, a target yet to be achieved. Although this may reduce the reliance upon overtime, shiftwork will remain. As well as improving the basic pay of health workers, shiftwork is essential if the community demands a comprehensive health-care service. However, there are ways to minimise the hardships. The Canadian Union of Public Employees suggests the following in its book *Health and Safety Hazards*:

- a shorter working week, extra days off and longer holidays;
- permanent or semi-permanent night shifts for as many workers who would find it convenient;
- providing as many services as possible for night staff, for example cafeterias and pleasant rest rooms;
- organising longer shift-patterns so that acclimatisation can occur.

By increasing worker participation in decision making some of the worst effects of hierarchical structures and job dissatisfaction may be overcome. The aim should be to introduce teamwork wherever possible, and to involve all levels of workers. Successful experiments along these lines have taken place already in Finland. This is how a hospital psychologist described the experiment:

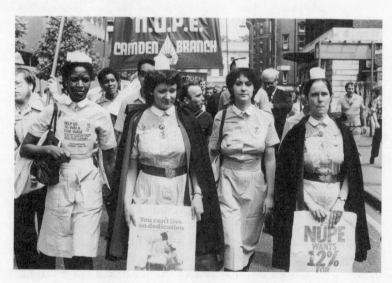

Protesting against low pay (courtesy Denis Doran).

Staff became more interested and more active and it seemed that role differences began to disappear. Everyone felt that they had a part to play in trying to cure patients. Work was done in small groups and soon the nursing staff started showing increased interest in reading trade journals and books.

In addition to this approach, consideration should be given to matching the skills of individuals with existing jobs where possible.

Finally, measures should be taken to improve the environment in which the work is done. Stress factors like heat, noise and light can readily be controlled. It is the responsibility of every shop steward to put improvement in the quality of life at the top of their bargaining list.

BACKPAIN

Contrary to what most people believe, backpain is not something only nurses suffer. Porters, ambulance crews, radiographers and other hospital workers run the risk of injuring their backs as well. Table 6.1 spells out this situation very clearly.

The overwhelming majority of back injuries happen during the lifting of patients. A further indication of the size of the problem is seen from a survey showing over 25 per cent of patients requiring lifting or lifting assistance. Almost half were geriatric patients while the others were in the medical, surgical and orthopaedic wards. Clearly, nurses and ambulance staff suffer a disproportionate number of accidents when lifting patients. A recent survey of nurses, published in 1981 (see the reference to Stubbs *et al.* at the end of this chapter), suggested about three-quarters of a million working days are lost each year through back injuries and around one in six nurses said handling patients was the cause of their backpain. Using these figures, it has been estimated that some forty thousand nurses are off sick with backpain every year.

Backpain is a problem affecting the whole working population; the DHSS estimate that more than $11\frac{1}{2}$ million working days are lost each year through back injuries. The cost to the country in terms of the health of workers is enormous. Many of the reasons for lifting accidents can be summed up as the failure to give training, lifting aids and safe systems of work.

Table 6.1 Summary of accidents involving the lifting or supporting of patients in the health services reported to the Factory Inspectorate during the second quarter of 1982

Occupation	Number of accidents	%
Nurse	664	52.44
Auxiliary nurse	258	20.37
Community nurse	13	1.02
Ambulance staff	199	15.71
Porter	31	2.44
Radiographer	3	0.23
Other	93	7.34
Not known	5	0.39
Totals	1266	100.

Biology of the Spine

The human spine is made up of twenty-four individual bones known as vertebrae. These form a column between the skull and pelvis. In fact it is common to find some men with twenty-five vertebrae and some women with twenty-three. Successive vertebrae are separated by pads of fibrous tissue called intervertebral discs beside which the spinal cord runs. Discs may be thought of as shock absorbers, their thickness varying according to whether a person is standing, sitting, stooping forward or supporting weights. Discs readily absorb water from the surrounding tissue fluids and swell. During the day they become dehydrated through activity but, at night they reabsorb water, hence the variation in height between evening and morning. Discs and vertebrae are all linked together by a complex pattern of muscles and ligaments. The result is a spine with a gentle curve referred to as posture.

Medical Causes of Backpain

The medical causes of backpain can be divided into four basic groups: primary, secondary, referred and psychosomatic.

Primary backpain

The tissues of the spine are supplied with nerves whose endings react to any kind of irritation. If these tissues are disturbed by frequent or heavy lifting, primary backpain occurs; it is often severe and is often felt in the buttocks and backs of the thighs. It commonly arises when a disc between vertebrae moves and touches the tissues of the spine. In these cases delays of 24 hours or more are not uncommon. This condition is often associated with severe pain in the leg. Another survey of nurses, published in 1979, found that about one third with backpain also complained of leg pain.

Secondary backpain

If the nerves supplying the spine are compressed or stretched so that the blood supply and conductivity are affected, secondary backpain occurs. Similarly it also occurs if the nerves are irritated. Generally this condition arises through disc degeneration and may allow pain to stay unchecked.

Referred backpain

Diseases of the abdomen or pelvis rather than lifting operations are responsible for this.

Psychosomatic backpain

This condition is rare and may arise in cases of depression, acute anxiety or hysteria. However, it is more likely to accompany an organic cause of pain. Workers suffering from chronic back pain often become depressed, and should be treated with sympathy.

Causes of Backpain at Work

Causes of backpain at work fall into three broad categories, as follows.

Spells of lifting

Backpain occurs where lifting is not a regular part of the job; it is similar to that experienced by a person after the first sports game of the season.

Postural stress

Bending down, like the jib of a crane, for a long time is a familiar cause of this. After straightening up a person very often experiences some discomfort and stiffness. Where work involves regular bending down, damage to the spinal tissues can occur. Sometimes nurses experience this pain when asked to hold a patient's limb or a piece of equipment in an awkward position.

Back injuries

Among workers this is the commonest cause of backpain, occurring where the lifting strength of a person is less than or equal to the actual lifting forces required. In this situation, a back injury is more likely to happen. Similarly, if a person feels that the loads are heavier than usual then back injuries can occur. Some researchers have found a link between pain and a feeling of undue effort among nurses.

Prevention of Backpain

There is no simple solution to this but an understanding of the causes and effects of backpain suggests two basic approaches have the best chance of success: first, improvement of the working environment within which the lifting is done; second, a wider recognition of the importance of training, safe systems of work and lifting aids. We can now look at these approaches in more detail.

Working environment

Any lifting task is likely to be dangerous if there is insufficient space, poor lighting, slippery or wet floors or other obstructions in the work area. Safety reps should look at the design of the workplace taking these factors into account; in a hospital ward where patient handling occurs this may involve the layout of beds, screens, ward furniture, baths and toilets to allow the use of mobile hoists. Other measures like the introduction of adjustable-height beds ease the problems. Similarly, manual handling tasks are made easier by having sufficiently wide work areas to allow manoeuvrability, floors free of grease and non-slip, store cupboards and shelves at the correct height. Minor changes, costing little money, can readily reduce the causes of backache.

Training

Employers have a legal obligation under the Health and Safety at Work Act to provide training for their workers. In practice either very little training is given or none at all. Surveys on training in patient handling by the unions COHSE, GMBATU and NUPE found a wide variation in practice between hospitals. Porters and auxiliary nurses were found to receive little formal training, and nurses received on average about three hours' teaching. In many instances no training was given in the use of hoists and lifts. Equally, training in the manual handling of loads is not much better, as government statistics demonstrate, with around 75,000 accidents every year.

Of course, the answer is training, including advice on the likely hazards, use of lifting aids and the variation in people's capacity to lift. To be of any benefit, practical as well as theoretical training must be given and should be long enough to develop the various lifting techniques into an everyday routine. Before lifting patients or loads insist upon proper training, or else you will become another back injury statistic.

Safe systems of work

The simplest way to avoid these problems is to carry out a thorough investigation of the lifting task: what aids and equipment are available, layout of the work area, likely risks and adequacy of training. The aim must be to reduce physical lifting to a minimum and to make sure as many risks as possible have been removed.

Of course, part of setting up a safe system of work means deciding on how many workers are needed for any lifting task. For instance, using the shoulder lift to move a patient requires two nurses of equal size. When deciding on staffing levels account should be taken of:

- absences due to sickness and injury;
- skills and experience of available staff;
- the availability of staff in nearby locations, for example wards, to offer help.

At all times there should be sufficient staff available to lift safely.

Lifting aids

If lifting accidents are to be reduced, more use should be made of mechanical lifting aids. A large range of lifting equipment is available for handling all manner of patients, but is often not used. Nurses rarely receive adequate training and the design of hospitals frequently prevents their efficient use. Very often lifting aids are not employed simply because they are too time-consuming, but this should not deter anyone from using them: a back injury can remain with you for the rest of your life. Similarly, wherever a load requires lifting, consideration should be given to the possibility of handling it mechanically.

Weight Limits

The maximum weight a person can safely lift very much depends on their age, sex, state of health and, of course, training. Age is an obvious factor but the sex of an individual is equally important; researchers have found that the lifting capacity of women is about two-thirds that of men. The health of a person lifting should always be taken into consideration, since permanent or temporary disabilities often impair the ability to lift. Equally, training is essential because it helps the body to overcome fatigue. Taking all these factors into consideration, American researchers reckon that nine out of ten adults can lift 16 kg (35 lb) and that eight out of ten can safely lift up to 34 kg (75 lb). But this is only a guide since it assumes that the lifting takes place in ideal conditions; it does not eliminate the risk of injury. Remember, a strained back can mean an injury for life.

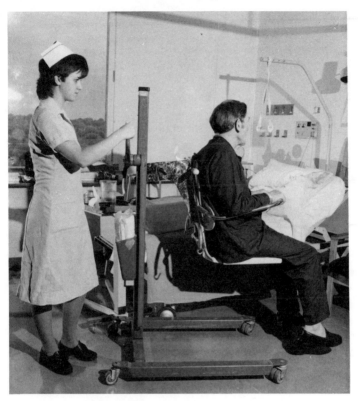

Using a lifting aid (photo: A. Nicola).

SAFETY CHECKLISTS

Stress

Do any staff work excessive overtime?
Is anyone on shiftwork complaining of poor sleep, bad digestion or
  depression?
Do staff on shiftwork complain of family or social problems?
Do individuals find their jobs challenging and stimulating?
Is too much responsibility making anyone feel ill?
Are individuals' workloads too great?
Are there frequent conflicts with superiors?

Are conflicting instructions frequently given by different supervisors?

Are working conditions satisfactory?

Do any of the staff complain of hypertension, heart disease or peptic ulcers?

Is anyone complaining of anxiety, fatigue, depression or aggression?

What steps have been taken to reduce stress?

Backpain

Do staff complain of backpain?

Is the workplace safe to lift in?

Is practical and theoretical training given to all staff who lift patients or equipment?

Are lifting aids readily available?

Is everyone taught how to use lifting aids?

Have safe systems of work been devised for all lifting tasks?

If so, is all lifting kept to a minimum?

Are staffing levels adequate to cope with lifting?

Has any consideration been given to the maximum weight an individual can lift?

REFERENCES

Backpain

Health and Safety Commission (1982). *Health and Safety (Manual Handling of Loads) Regulations and Guidance (1982)*

P. Lloyd, C. Osborne, C. Tarling and D. Troup (1981). *The Handling of Patients*. Shears, Basingstoke

S.T. Pheasant (1980). The biomechanisms of the human spine. *Proceedings of the Conference on the Prevention of Back Pain in Nursing*. Nursing Practice Research Unit, Northwick Park Hospital, Harrow, Middlesex

D.A. Stubbs, P.W. Buckle, M.P. Hudson, D.M. Rivers, and C.J. Warringham (1981). *Back Pain in the Nursing Profession, Part*

1. Materials Handling Research Unit, University of Surrey, Guildford

D. Troup (1980). The causes of back pain at work, and the mechanisms of back injury. *Proceedings of the Conference on the Prevention of Back Pain in Nursing*

Working Group on Lifting of Patients in the Health Service (1982). *Report*. A private communication to the Health Services Advisory Committee of the Health and Safety Commission

Stress

C. Bradley and T. Cox (1978). *Stress at Work*. Macmillan, Basingstoke and London, ch.4

P. Brooks (1980). Stress at Work: 2, 'The tension of the bells'. *Health and Safety at Work*, vol.3, No.2, October 1980

M. Bryan (1976). Hazards to the Health and Safety of Hospital Employees. Public Services International, Feltham, Middlesex

C. Mackay and T. Cox (1978). *Stress at Work*. Macmillan, Basingstoke and London, ch.7

N. McDonald and M. Doyle (1981). *The Stresses of Work*. Nelson, London, chh. 2, 4 and 5

H. Murrell (1978). *Work Stress and Mental Strain*. Work Research Unit, Department of Employment, London

7.   Sexual Harassment and Assaults

SEXUAL HARASSMENT

Sexual harassment at work is nothing new for women workers. They have had to put up with the unwelcome attention of men in the past for fear of being spoilsports. Of course, those who do it say it livens up the daily routine of work. After all, they say, it's nothing more than harmless fun, only natural when men and women work together, but that is not a view shared by most women. Sex in the office, factory or hospital, the subject of lurid cracks by music hall comedians, is now a joke that has long since lost its humour.

Trade unions like NALGO, GMBATU, and NUPE say that sexual harassment at work is an issue which affects the rights of working women. But many trade unionists feel it is a fuss about nothing. However, a confidential survey by the Alfred Marks Employment Agency showed that women felt sexual harassment was a major problem; over half those who were victims of it felt strongly enough about it to leave their jobs. Again, a survey in the magazine *Cosmopolitan* found that over 95 per cent of the women participating had experienced sexual harassment of one kind or another. Of the men who replied to the survey, over half frankly admitted that they made sexual advances to women colleagues and went on to say that they thought most women actually did not object. The survey also showed that being the object of sexual harassment is not confined to young, attractive women but is also experienced by women of all ages, shapes and sizes, and that all kinds of men, including those in their sixties, are willing harassers.

Certainly, sexual harassment is a problem in the health services; for many women it has become an everyday occurrence. A woman will have no difficulty deciding whether unwelcome attentions are being paid to her. For instance, the harasser is likely to put his arms round her waist, insist on kissing her, may even go as far as phoning her at home and, of course, will inevitably suggest that they sleep together. Most men will tolerate this behaviour by their workmates as long as their wife or daughter is not the subject of a harasser's attention.

As we said earlier this is a trade union issue, so what exactly is sexual harassment and what can be done about it?

What Is Sexual Harassment?

In society men are in a dominant position, exercising power over women in the labour market. Limited job opportunities, high unemployment and low wages combine to keep women in this vulnerable position. Against this background, sexual harassment can be defined as sexual advances which may threaten a woman worker's job or health. Sexual advances made by men with authority can threaten the job security, career prospects and job satisfaction of women workers. In this situation women are not judged on their abilities and qualifications for a job but as sex objects.

Most victims of sexual harassment experience suggestive remarks and looks, physical contact like touching or pinching, demands for sexual favours and occasionally physical assault, sometimes ending in rape. Often these accompany threats to a woman's job or career prospects if she is unwilling to co-operate. An article in the *New Statesman* by a woman working for a theatrical costumiers described how her life was made intolerable by her employer's repeated sexual advances, and that when she rejected him he gave her less interesting work, forcing her to leave.

Men often view their behaviour as harmless fun and complain that women don't have a sense of humour or take the fun out of life. But sexual harassment is very different from flirtation, which relies on mutual consent; it is, rather, unwanted sexual advances accompanied by promises, abuse or threats.

What Are the Effects?

Anger is not the only emotion that sexual harassment causes. Victims suffer tension, anxiety, fear and frustration. The more often this happens the worse problems may become, often appearing as headaches, indigestion, ulcers and other nervous disorders. Extreme harassment can also cause serious depression and despair. The Canadian Union of Public Employees found that some cases were so serious that the women had to be admitted to hospital. Of course, in the most extreme cases there is the risk of physical injury.

As well as the health risks, the victim's ability to do her job is in jeopardy. The situation can become so bad that her employer may question her ability to do the job, and may decide to sack her. If this happens, she may find that her employer threatens her future job prospects by giving bad references. Matters are frequently made much worse if the woman leaves her job as a result of sexual harassment. Social Security officers often don't accept this as a satisfactory reason for leaving, and may deprive her of unemployment benefit for six weeks. But quitting a job is not something many women can risk doing.

What Can the Union Do?

Tackling sexual harassment is a trade union issue, and not one that should be left to the individual. It is a health and safety problem that affects the health and general well-being of women. Where this unwelcome behaviour arises women members should be able to turn to their union for advice and assistance. The role of the union in this situation is to ensure that the employer gives a commitment that behaviour of this kind will not be tolerated and that prompt action will be taken to stop it whenever it happens.

As a first step we suggest that the following agreement, drawn up by the Equal Pay and Opportunity Campaign (EPOC) as guidelines for trade unions and employers dealing with sexual harassment, is made the subject of a formal claim.

1. Sexual harassment of an employee by any other employee will not be tolerated.

2. Management will take prompt, corrective action upon becoming aware that incidents involving sexual harassment have taken place.
3. Sexual harassment will be grounds for disciplinary action.
4. Supervisors have a duty to maintain their workplace free from sexual harassment and intimidation.
5. Employees subjected to sexual harassment should report such conduct to their supervisor.
6. Supervisors should immediately report to a specified person any complaints of sexual harassment.
7. Management's policy and the procedure to be followed will be given to employees as part of their training and induction programmes.

Once management has accepted sexual harassment as a problem and it is part of the collective agreement, grievances can be taken under the normal procedure. Because of the embarrassing nature of this problem and the need to deal with it confidentially and speedily, a special grievance procedure may be thought more appropriate. A simple two-stage procedure is probably sufficient; at the first stage the complaint should be heard by a committee comprising of three women: a trade unionist, a management representative and someone from the District Health Authority (DHA) as chair. The committee should hear the complaint within ten working days from the time it is lodged. Their decision should be binding on both parties but, in the event of either of them being dissatisfied with it, there should be a right of appeal to the DHA. Again the committee should comprise only women members of the DHA and the complaint should be heard within twenty working days. In this way the often embarrassing nature of sexual harassment complaints can be handled with tact.

On a more general note, the local union branch should do as follows:

1. Make members aware of the problem of sexual harassment at work by encouraging discussion of this at branch meetings, writing articles and letters for the branch newsletter and arranging special meetings on this topic.
2. Ensure that sexual harassment is treated as a serious threat to job security and individual rights.

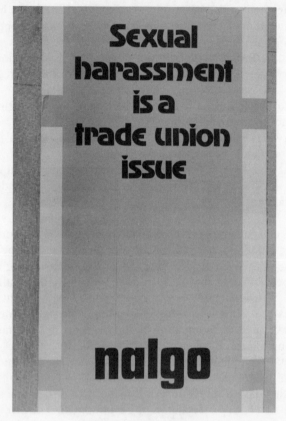

**Union pamphlet on
sexual harassment.**

3. Encourage shop stewards to be available to advise members on
   how to deal with the situation if sexually harassed. In particular
   the steward should:
   - listen sympathetically to a complaint of sexual harassment
     (often, victims find it embarrassing to report the incident, so
     the steward's role is to reassure them);
   - find out if other women are victims of the same harasser;
   - encourage the victim to keep a diary of incidents of harass-
     ment, including details of time, place and any witnesses;

- where the harasser is unaware that his behaviour is offensive, make him aware of his actions, and the possible consequences;
- discuss with management ways of dealing with the problem, pointing out that it is not satisfactory to solve the problem simply by transferring the victim to another department, unless she agrees; it should be the harasser and not the victim who is moved.

4. Consider designating a member of the branch as a contact for sexual harassment complaints, preferably a woman. This person would have a similar role to that of the shop steward on these matters.

5. Support members subject to sexual harassment through the grievances procedure and, if necessary, in legal action.

Of course, if the harasser is a colleague and union member, he may seek the support of the union, but no one should let this deter her from complaining about sexual harassment. Unions will judge each case on its merits. In their excellent pamphlet *Sexual Harassment at Work* Ann Sedley and Melissa Benn describe how a union official can help in this situation.

In November 1981, the Head Chef in a canteen of a major engineering company was dismissed for sexual harassment after two women had complained about his behaviour through their shop steward. As the man was a member of the Transport and General Workers Union, TGWU, he sought help from his District Officer, who agreed to attend his appeal hearing. The man's sacking was upheld and he asked for help in progressing an application of unfair dismissal to an industrial tribunal. However, the District Officer felt that the appeal had revealed clear evidence of sexual harassment of the two women. Also, all women working in the canteen wanted the company to take action.

The District Officer was willing to advise the man of his rights and help him make an application to a tribunal but would not do anything more for him. Although the TGWU have no policy on sexual harassment, he believed the existing policy on equal opportunity was clear and that the company was obliged to act against the man whose behaviour was so intolerable that he was forcing women out of employment. It is clear that such behaviour was 'gross misconduct' which entitled the company to dismiss him.'

What Can the Victim Do?

Sexual harassment is not a problem that will go away if the victim ignores it; harassers persist unless something is done about it. Unfortunately, many women think that they are somehow to blame for this unwarranted attention. In her article in the journal *The Leveller*, Jane Root quotes the case of a young woman approached by a hospital porter in her first job who said, 'I was young and naïve and automatically assumed that I had encouraged him in some way. Ashamed and embarrassed, I left the job several weeks early.' Many women have had similar experiences, so anyone who is a victim should not ignore it, but should do something about it.

As a first step, she should tell the harasser to stop, making it clear that his advances are uninvited. Sometimes it will help her to ask a friend or colleague to come with her when confronting him. At the same time she should discuss the problem with other women in her workplace to find out if the harasser behaves in a similar manner to them. If telling the harasser to stop does not work then she should approach her shop steward and seek his/her help to deal with the harasser. She should keep a diary of all incidents of harassment so that a case can be built up against him. At the same time, she should keep a record of her work activities because harassers often claim that a poor work record is the reason for sacking their victims when, in fact, the reason is that the employee will not comply with their sexual advances. This way she will avoid any attempt at victimisation. At the same time the shop steward should also be taking measures to stop the harasser. As we said earlier, the harasser will not go away if his victim simply ignores him so she must not feel guilty or embarrassed about taking action to stop him. Harassers will find all manner of excuses to justify their behaviour to the victim (her dress is provocative, her attitude invites sexual advances and so on) but she should not let this deter her. Sexual harassment is a flagrant abuse of power over women and must be vigorously resisted.

Of course, it is also possible to take cases of sex discrimination to an industrial tribunal (IT). In March 1982 Julie Hyatt, an office worker, complained to a tribunal about her employer's continuous sexual advances, ranging from being slapped on the bottom to her manager pushing himself against her, and was awarded over £900 compensation for unfair dismissal. In her *Office Workers' Survival Handbook* Marianne Craig quotes the case of an eighteen-year-old typist, Victoria Stevens, who won a case of unfair dismissal at Birmingham Industrial Tribunal in 1980. Her employer made repeated advances, but when she complained she was promptly sacked. However, we feel that going to an industrial tribunal should be treated as a last resort. Very few people succeed in their applications to ITs, and even less get reinstatement when they claim unfair dismissal. Instead, fight sexual harassment through your union.

Sexual harassment is not a new problem for women; it has a long history. But now women are taking positive action against this aggressive male behaviour. It will take time to change society's attitudes towards women, and meanwhile unions must take up this issue and actively campaign to eliminate sexual harassment from the workplace. Safety representatives and shop stewards have a very important role to play if this campaign is to succeed. Sexual harassment is not only an economic issue but also a health and safety matter. Remember, any kind of sexual advance, if it is unwelcome, threatens a woman's job as well as her health and general well-being.

ASSAULTS ON STAFF

Despite what most people believe, violence to staff in the health service is a persistent problem. A NUPE survey over a two-year period, 1976–8, brought to light 116 assaults in general hospitals. A similar TUC survey in 1976–7 uncovered 151 assaults, many of them unprovoked. Victims suffered bites, scratches, fractured ribs and even broken limbs. In one incident an ambulanceman was knocked unconscious and, in another, a nurse was nearly strangled. There are horrifying stories of knives, razors and chairs being used as weapons.

The evidence which exists points to assaults happening regularly in three situations. First, at casualty departments, especially late on a Thursday, Friday or Saturday night: see the case of Robert in Chapter 1. Figures for these incidents show that the majority happen at inner-city hospitals in places like Birmingham, Liverpool, London and Glasgow. Second, attacks by psychiatric patients are all too commonplace. Finally, attacks on nurses in hospital grounds are happening more and more frequently, sometimes ending in rape.

Employers have a duty under section 2(1) of the Health and Safety at Work Act to take steps to safeguard the safety of their workers. It is reasonable to interpret this duty as protection from foreseeable risk of assault by patients, relatives or friends with whom they come into contact in the course of their work. It is equally clear, however, that many employers have not considered problems of violence to their staff within the context of the Act.

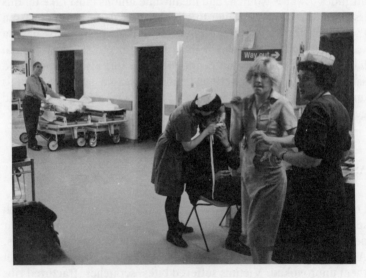

A typical Friday night in the casualty department of an inner-city hospital (photo: A. Nicola).

In 1976, the DHSS issued a circular, *The Management of Violent or Potentially Violent Patients*, advising health authorities to provide staff training to deal with these situations and to set up a comprehensive reporting system. Despite this guidance, NUPE found almost everywhere that reporting procedures were unsatisfactory and that training programmes were virtually nonexistent, although a few hospitals had produced some written material for nurses dealing with violent patients. We now look at how to deal with these incidents.

What Can Be Done About Assaults?

The main things which can help are as follows:

Security staff

As already mentioned, casualty staff at inner-city hospitals run the risk of being assaulted by patients and visitors alike. Because these situations can be very violent we would argue that fully trained hospital security staff should be on call. At the present time negotiations are taking place between the health service unions and the DHSS over this proposal. As usual, there is no money available to carry out these proposals. Here again successive governments have failed to make extra money available for health and safety matters, so any health and safety problems which cost money have to compete with other demands upon health authority budgets. Very often, the choice is between spending money on health and safety and spending it on patient care. Faced with this choice, the dedication of health workers ensures that patients' needs are met first. The DHSS are aware of this dilemma, and don't press for more funds to cover health and safety.

Protection

There is no shortage of horrifying accounts of assaults on nurses as they walk between the nurses' home and hospital. All too often the pathway is unlit, isolated from the main hospital buildings and infrequently used. At least three things can be done to make paths safer:

- installation of path lighting;
- regular security patrols, especially at night;
- provision of hand-held alarms.

Staffing

In many cases the only way of dealing with violent situations in hospital is with extra staff. But cuts in public expenditure have meant that understaffing is widespread in the health service, so staff are left on their own to deal with violent situations. This is frequently the case in psychiatric hospitals. In its report on *Assaults on NHS Staff* the TUC describes an incident of a nursing assistant left alone on night duty in a psychiatric ward, who was attacked by a patient using a detachable cot side as a weapon. She suffered severe spinal damage and never worked again. Clearly, wherever there is a danger of assault, staffing levels should be adequate to cope.

Alarms

In the last resort some means of summoning immediate assistance is required. An alarm system which attracts the attention of staff in the vicinity, or alerts a central control, possibly the porter's lodge, may be the answer. However, this is no substitute for proper staffing levels or, in the case of inner-city hospitals, internal security staff.

Training

This is important if staff are to cope with violence. Management have a responsibility under section 2(2)(c) of the Health and Safety at Work Act to provide training and supervision for staff who may be at risk from assault. Training should be extended to all health service workers, including ancillary staff, who come into contact with the public. The core of any course should show how to deal with a personal attack.

What Can You Do If Assaulted?

There are several things you can do:

- call for assistance, or ask the nearest person to summon help;
- remain calm and do not react to abusive remarks;
- don't attempt to restrain the person unless assistance is available;
- if, as a member of ambulance staff, you come into contact with a potentially violent patient, don't attempt to move him if it is a single-manned vehicle; get assistance;
- make sure you report every incident to management.

Compensation

For workers injured as a result of assault at work, there are a number of sources of income and compensation. Sick pay is the most common; others include NHS injury benefit and criminal injuries compensation. We look at these in some detail now.

Sick pay

Previously, anyone absent from work because of an accident could claim Industrial Injury Benefit but this has now been abolished. Instead, workers should receive sick pay from their employers for the first eight weeks absent and then sickness and invalidity benefit for longer periods. Sick pay is paid at a standard rate, and is taxable. At the time of introducing these proposals the government also changed the sick note scheme. Now, if you are absent because of injury for less than eight days you don't need a sick note, but require a self-certificate after three days absent.

NHS Injury Allowance

All health service workers are covered by this scheme which is payable to anyone off work because of an injury. What the scheme does is guarantee a minimum income of 85 per cent of your weekly wage after taking sick pay into account. To qualify, a worker must be on sick leave with reduced or no pay as a result of the injury.

Normally, on returning to work payment of this allowance stops but, if as a result of the injury, a worker's earning ability is permanently reduced by more than 10 per cent or, if he has to give up work, then he is entitled to a permanent allowance. This allowance is guaranteed for life and, if he gives up work, a lump sum is also paid out. But any damages or compensation awarded are taken into account when working out entitlement to the allowance. Table 7.1 sets out the actual allowance and lump-sum entitlements as a percentage of final pay.

And, if a worker's earning ability deteriorates further then the permanent allowance can be re-assessed. Where death occurs, a regular allowance is payable to the widow and certain dependents to top up any existing NHS pension to a percentage of the worker's final pay, as shown in table 7.2.

Table 7.1 Permanent injury allowance entitlements

| Reduction of earning ability | Guaranteed income (including scheme pension and Social Security benefits) | | | | Lump sum |
| | Employment | | | | |
	Less than 5 years	5 years and over but less than 15 years	15 years and over but less than 25 years	25 years and over	
More than 10% but not more than 25%	15%	30%	45%	60%	12½%
More than 25% but not more than 50%	40%	50%	60%	70%	25%
More than 50% but not more than 75%	65%	70%	75%	80%	37½%
More than 75%	85%	85%	85%	85%	50%

Table 7.2   Regular allowances payable on death

Widow	45%
Each of the first 4 children	10% if there is a widow or 20% if there is no widow
Each incapacitated adult child	20% if there is a surviving parent or 45% if there is no surviving parent
Each incapacitated adult child	20% if there is a surviving parent or 45% if there is no surviving parent
One dependent parent	20% if there is a widow or 45% if there is no widow

If a lump sum has not already been paid out under the scheme then a lump sum of 25 per cent of final pay is given. The permanent allowances are inflation-proof but temporary allowances are only given similar protection for people aged 55 and over.

Criminal Injuries Compensation Scheme

This scheme provides lump-sum compensation from government funds for anyone injured as a result of a violent crime, or the prevention (or attempted prevention) of an offence. It was set up in 1964, and pays out around £11 million every year. Even victims of assault by psychiatric patients can claim. Over half the awards in 1977–8 came into the range £100–£400. Claims are settled by the Criminal Injuries Compensation Board (CICB), which is composed of legally qualified persons appointed by the Home Secretary in consultation with the Lord Chancellor. Compensation is assessed in two parts, general damages for pain and loss of pleasure caused by the injury and special damages for any financial losses. The Board will not deal with claims where damages are likely to be less than £150. However, there is no maximum limit.

Compensation from this source, however, does not stop an action for damages through the courts, but any amounts recovered are deducted from criminal-injuries compensation. Similarly, the Board is obliged to deduct any Social Security payments and any monies paid out under the National Health Service insurance scheme. So far the experience of some unions has been that CICB awards often fall below the level of court awards in similar cases.

To qualify for this scheme the following information has to be given:

- the time and place of the incident;
- a brief account of the incident;
- details of action taken;
- details of injury to staff and/or patients.

Further information about the scheme can be found in a leaflet *Crimes of Violence: A Guide to the Compensation Scheme* obtainable from the Criminal Injuries Compensation Board, 10–12 Russell Square, London WC1B 5EN.

Union Benefit Schemes

Nearly all unions operate a benefit scheme whereby members are entitled to receive benefit for accidents at work as long as medical evidence of incapacity is produced. As well as this, benefit is usually paid for loss of sight, for loss of a limb or limbs and for fatal accidents. Full details of these benefits can be found in the union's rule book.

SAFETY CHECKLIST

Sexual Harassment

Do any women complain of unwelcome attention from men?
Do any women suffer tension, anxiety, fear or frustration as a result?

Do any women find their jobs affected as a result?
Do management have a policy for dealing with sexual harassment?
Is there a sexual harassment grievance procedure?
Has your union a policy on sexual harassment?
Are union leaflets on this problem available?
Are articles on sexual harassment appearing in your union's national and local journals?
Are shop stewards and safety reps able to give advice?
Has your union given advice on how to deal with a harasser?

Assaults

Do any of the staff complain of being assaulted?
Where do the assaults happen?
Are security staff on call?
Are staffing levels adequate to cope?
Are hand-held alarms available?
Are the grounds adequately lit?
Are the grounds regularly patrolled?
Is everyone told how to deal with an assault?
What advice has been given on compensation?

REFERENCES

S. Attenborough (1981). *Sexual Harassment at Work*. National Union of Provincial Government Employees (Canada), 204-2841 Riverside Drive, Ottawa, Ontario, K1V, 8N4
M. Craig (1981). *Office Workers' Survival Handbook*. British Society for Social Responsibility in Society in Science, 9 Poland Street, London W1.
J. McIntosh (1982). Sexual harassment—you tell us, it's not a joke. *Cosmopolitan*, Oct. 1982
National Association of Local Government Officers (1982). *Sexual Harassment is a Trade Union Issue*. NALGO, 1 Mabledon Place, London WC1H 9AJ

J. Root (1981). Sexual harassment at work. *The Leveller*, 17 Apr. 1981

M. Rubenstein (1981). When the office Romeo violates the law. *Personnel Management*, Oct. 1981

A. Sedley and M. Benn (1982). *Sexual Harassment at Work*. National Council for Civil Liberties, Russell Press, London

8. Preventing Accidents and Ill Health

LEGISLATION BEFORE 1974

Today it is commonplace for any trade union conference to make demands for greater safety at work; this is all part of the struggle for better working conditions. But trade unions have been pressing for improvements in health and safety law since the last century. It was in 1833 that the Whig government under pressure passed the first effective Factory Act, which regulated the hours of work of children and young persons, and ended the practice of employing children under nine except in silk mills.* However, only four factory inspectors were appointed to enforce the new law. Most employers were quick to condemn this legislation as a wanton and ruinous interference in business and soon found ways round it. The 1847 Factory Act was to receive an even more stormy reception; employers strongly objected to the limit set in the number of hours women and youths could work in factories.

The rapid growth of the factory system meant that there were hundreds of thousands of workers not protected by the law. Although progress was slow the Factory Acts were extended during the period 1860–1900 to include many dangerous and unhealthy trades. During this time, workers in the coal industry achieved the appointment of their own Workmen's Inspectors. Similarly, railway workers won the appointment of two 'assistant inspectors' from their own ranks. Other groups of workers were making similar demands because they did not trust the government inspectors. The fight for healthier and safer working conditions continued into this century. Between 1906 and 1943 no less

*Some historians call Peel's Act of 1802 the first Factory Act but it was only a new provision of the Poor Law. In fact, all it did was end the practice of employing children under nine in cotton factories. But there were no inspectors to enforce the Act, so it was generally ignored by employers and parents alike.

than seven Acts dealing with health and safety found their way onto the statute book. But it was not until 1924 that the TUC began demanding the right for workers to have some control over their working conditions; until then they had a poor track record.

By 1952 the TUC was calling for the appointment of trade union safety representatives, a demand that was in response to the growing number of accidents in industry. Between 1950 and 1973, the year before the Health and Safety at Work Act, over 15,000 workers lost their lives, and this excludes those who died from occupational diseases contracted earlier in their working lives ; many occupational diseases are not notifiable and do not form part of the Factory Inspectorate's statistics. During this period there was a growing dissatisfaction with the existing health and safety laws, in particular among the eight million workers in the public sector, including the health service, who were not covered by any of the existing legislation. NUPE and other public-sector unions had been agitating for legislation to protect their members.

In 1968, under pressure from the trade union movement, the then Labour government set up the Safety and Health at Work Committee, under the chairmanship of Lord Robens, to examine the problem; its conclusions (Cmnd 5034; HMSO) were given to the Conservative government in 1972 but they were defeated at the polls before enacting new legislation. The return of a Labour government in 1974, however, led to the Health and Safety at Work Act. With the passing of this Act, safety law was extended to about eight million people who had previously been outside its scope, and those now covered included people working in places like hospitals. Unlike previous safety laws, the HASAW Act did not deal with specific hazards; instead, it attempted to cope in a general way with all health and safety problems in the workplace. The aim of this approach was to allow safety law to keep pace with the rapid changes in technology and the new hazards that they brought into the workplace.

THE HEALTH AND SAFETY AT WORK ACT ETC. 1974

Employers' Duties to Employees

The act imposes eight main duties on an employer, namely to:

- provide and maintain all plant including machinery, equipment and systems of work that are safe and without risk to health (section 2(2)(a));
- remove any risks when using, handling, storing and transporting articles and substances (section 2(2)(b));
- provide information, instructions, training and supervision (section 2(2)(c));
- provide a safe workplace with safe access and exit from the building(s) (section 2(2)(d));
- provide a safe working environment (section 2(2)(e));
- provide adequate welfare facilities (section 2(2)(e));
- provide protective clothing or equipment free of charge when required to do so under specific regulations (section 9);
- provide a health and safety policy which must be brought to the attention of all employees (section 2(3)).

We now look at two of these duties in detail to see what they actually mean.

The first duty states that an employer must provide and maintain a safe workplace and systems of work. Therefore health authorities have a legal duty to maintain the standards of their hospital kitchens at an adequate level. In practice, this means they must replace unsafe equipment and make regular inspections of the kitchens to ensure everything is safe. Of course, when buying new equipment like stoves they must take into account safety features and not just the cost. Equally, they must take into account the worker's views before new purchases are made.

The third duty listed is one of the most important placed on the employer: the provision of adequate training and information. This means that every worker must be properly trained for the job they are doing, which includes the provision of information about hazards and how to avoid them. Employers should provide training on the particular dangers of their workplace. This should supplement (and not replace) the TUC training course for safety reps. This means, for instance, that health authorities should tell operating theatre staff about the dangers of waste anaesthetic gases. One way of making certain employers do this is for workers to refuse to do any jobs for which they have not been trained, or about any associated hazards of which they have not been given enough information.

Employers' Duties to Other People

Employers have a responsibility to make sure that the public are not put at risk by anything done in connection with their business. For instance, both patients and visitors in hospital must not be exposed to any risks.

Duties of Employees

Workers as well as employers have certain duties under the Act. These are:

- to take reasonable care of themselves and others (section 7(a));
- to co-operate with the employer so that he can meet his duties under the Act in making the workplace safe (section 7(b));
- not to misuse anything provided to make the workplace safer (section 8).

But this does not mean that the responsibility for health and safety is shared equally between the workers and the employer. On the contrary, it simply means that employees may be prosecuted if they misuse equipment or smoke in non-smoking areas; however, it is unlikely that most workers would risk their lives for a quick fag!

Duties of Manufacturers and Suppliers

These include:

- making sure that articles or substances they produce are safe and without risk to health;
- carrying out tests and examinations on them to confirm they are safe;
- providing information on how to use their products;
- researching into any risks that may be associated with them (section 6).

Although your workplace may be reasonably safe, a new piece of equipment or a new chemical could easily put the health of you and your workmates at risk. The duties just listed are designed to stop this happening by ensuring that in the first place the manufacturer has thoroughly tested the piece of equipment or chemical and that adequate operating instructions have been provided. So make certain that the manufacturers' or suppliers' safety instructions have been handed out.

'Reasonably Practicable'

Now, the general duties of employers to their employees and others, as set out above, have an important qualification to them. Under section (2) of the Act it states:

> It should be the general duty of every employer to ensure, as far as is reasonably practicable, the health, safety and welfare at work of all his employees.

So employers need do only what is 'as far as is reasonably practicable' to protect the health, safety and welfare of their workers. This turns out to be a very handy get-out for many employers simply because it means that risk is weighed against the cost. If the risk is high and the cost of removing it low then, of course, it is reasonably practicable. On the other hand, if the risk is low but the cost of removing it is high then it is not reasonably practicable, and an employer is justified in doing nothing about it. Of course, the risk may be low simply because no one has been hurt but that does not mean someone will not be seriously injured in the future as a result of not removing the risk.

Safety reps can deal with this problem in two ways. First, they can borrow standards from other sources to support their case that their proposals are reasonably practicable. For instance, suppose a safety rep is concerned about the ventilation and temperature in the hospital laundry. She or he can turn to sections 3 and 4 of the Factories Act 1961 for guidance on suitable standards. Although these legally apply only to factories there is nothing to stop her from borrowing them. Second, safety reps can tip the balance of risk and cost in favour of better production by finding out as much as possible about the real costs of removing the risk and the number of accidents that occur but are not reported. This means that safety reps will have to keep a record of all injuries, however minor, that occur in the workplace. One person fainting because of poor ventilation and high temperature may not be enough but if others are complaining of exhaustion and occasionally fainting, then a convincing case can be built up.

TRADE UNION SAFETY REPRESENTATIVES

Earlier we said that the election of safety representatives by workers was a long-standing union demand. On the passage of the Health and Safety at Work Act this became a reality. Unions were given the right to appoint safety representatives who have legal powers to challenge management's control over all matters affecting safety and health. Details of these rights are given in the Safety Representatives and Safety Committee Regulations along with a Code of Practice and Guidance Notes explaining how they operate in practice. In fact, it was 1978 before they became law simply because employers saw the Regulations as an erosion of the right to run their own businesses. Of course, many were aware of the impact safety representatives would have in improving conditions at work.

Who Can Be a Safety Rep?

The Regulations give unions the right to elect their own safety representatives at every workplace where they are recognised. Now a 'recognised' union is one which is accepted by the employer for the purposes of negotiations over pay and working conditions. However, a union must also be independent, by which we mean that it is not run or supported financially by the employer. In the Health Service, all TUC-affiliated unions like COHSE, NALGO, GMBATU and NUPE are independent and recognised.

When the Regulations first became law there was a debate among unions over who should be a safety rep. Basically, the argument was about whether existing workplace representatives like shop stewards should take on these additional responsibilities or whether members other than the stewards should become safety representatives. Those who took the view that shop stewards were the most suitable argued that health and safety improvements required employers to spend money and that reps with negotiating experience were needed. But, on the other hand, their opponents said, they already had sufficient to do and probably wouldn't have the time necessary to deal with safety problems. Most unions overcame these differences by adopting a flexible approach, allowing their members to decide what was the best way to deal with it in their particular workplace.

On the question 'Who can be a safety rep?' the Regulations specifically say the following.

- Anyone wishing to be a safety rep should normally have worked for their present employer for at least two years, or have had two years experience in similar work. Nevertheless, there are exceptional circumstances where these requirements may be waived — where, for example, there is a high turnover of staff.
- After the safety rep is elected their name and details of the group of workers they represent has to be given in writing to the employer.
- The safety rep stays in office unless the union tells the employer otherwise, in writing.

It is important that safety reps always reflect the views of their members. This is best achieved by ensuring safety reps are elected on a regular basis, and that there is a spot on the agenda of the branch meeting to report back.

How Many?

This is a difficult question to answer, especially since the Regulations give little guidance. Obviously, several factors, like the variety of jobs, workplace locations and shift systems, must be taken into account. Porters, for instance, probably require more safety reps than hospital gardeners simply because they work on a shift system. However, some idea of the total needed can be got from the number of shop stewards in the workplace. It is up to the union to decide on how many safety reps are required, and if there is any problem then the matter should be dealt with through the normal negotiating procedures.

Legal Liability

Workers may be deterred from standing as safety reps by the thought that they will run the risk of legal action if they either agree or do not object to action taken by the employer when dealing with a particular hazard. In fact, there is a specific safeguard in the Regulations which protects safety reps against prosecution, but this does not remove their legal responsibilities as employees. Like other workers they are obliged to take reasonable care and work with the employer as far as necessary to allow him to fulfil his legal health and safety duties.

Time Off and Training

Obviously, time off during working hours is essential if safety reps are to do their job properly. The Regulations specifically say that they are entitled to time off with pay to carry out their functions. If any employer refuses this, a complaint can be made to an industrial tribunal. In addition, make sure adequate time is given to complete inspection forms and write reports after inspections or investigations. Knowing the reluctance of many employers to concede time off for union duties, it will probably be necessary to negotiate the amount of time off.

It is as important to receive training as it is to have time off for safety rep's duties. Again, the Regulations say that employers must give safety reps time off with pay to take a basic training course. Since the purpose is to train safety reps as union officials, the training course must be approved by the TUC or the rep's union. Clearly, there would be a conflict of interest if the employer was to provide the training. Further training can be taken by safety reps to meet changes in work practice or relevant legislation. This will probably be given by the employer because it will deal with specific hazards in his workplace: for example, dealing with the problem of waste anaesthetic gases in operating theatres, or the risk of back injury from lifting patients.

Before you go off on a course as the newly elected safety rep, make sure the union has got approval from the employer for you to attend. Try and give a few weeks notice and let the employer see the course syllabus if he asks. Remember, attending a course shows you how to raise issues with the employer, spot hazards, write reports and encourage interest in health and safety among members.

What Safety Representatives Can Do

Under the Regulations safety reps have been given a number of important functions. These can be broken down as follows.

Formal inspections

A safeguard against accidents occurring is the right to inspect workplaces. As long as the employer has been told, safety reps can inspect their workplace:

- every three months;
- when there has been a substantial change in the conditions of work: this would include, for instance, the inspection of a refurbished operating theatre or the purchase of new floor polishers for the domestic staff;
- when new information has been published by the Health and Safety Commission (HSC) or Health and Safety Executive (HSE) which is relevant to the workplace. For example, the booklet on VDUs.

In many cases it may be felt that three months is far too long between inspections, so many unions have successfully negotiated inspections on a more frequent basis, for example monthly. Incidentally, employers can be present at these inspections if they wish, but discussions with workers can take place in private.

Investigation of dangerous occurrences and potential hazards

When dangerous occurrences happen safety reps have the right to investigate them. In technical jargon, a dangerous occurrence is an incident which has the potential to cause serious injury to employees or members of the public, although injury may not in fact have occurred. Put simply, a dangerous occurrence is nothing more than a near miss, but it is important to investigate these if accidents are to be prevented. An everyday example of this is the lifting of patients — many nurses are just not properly trained to lift the right way. Similarly, safety reps also have the right to investigate potential hazards. Again, a typical example is trailing leads in a ward or operating theatre — both have the potential to cause nasty accidents like broken arms or legs.

Investigation of accidents

Of course, accidents do happen and safety reps have the right to find out why, which is important if they are to be prevented from happening again. But, before actually carrying out an investigation you must make certain it is safe to do so. To get a picture of the events leading up to the accident you will probably need to ask these questions:

- What happened immediately before the accident?
- Were any of these events out of the ordinary?
- What happened straight after the accident?
- What instructions had been given?
- Was anyone supervising?
- Are there any legal requirements relating to the job?
- Were all house rules and regulations complied with?

To the answers should be added a general description of the working conditions including reference to such things as temperature, noise, space and any other relevant points. Often the real cause of the accident is masked by other apparent causes, so it may call for some detective work to identify it. As part of the investigation, take the names and addresses of all witnesses and, if possible, short signed statements as well. However, witnesses are not obliged either to answer any questions or to make any statements except to the Health and Safety inspector or, in the case of a fatal accident, to the Coroner, or in Scotland the Sheriff. If they refuse they need not give any reasons. Equally, some employers try to get statements from workers straight after the accident so they can shift the blame onto the injured person. Since most people are in a state of shock after an accident they should not give the employer any signed statements. Instead, an account of the accident should be put in the Accident Book and preferably not by the injured person.

Complaints

Safety reps have also been given the right to investigate complaints from members. Since it is impossible to inspect the workplace on a daily basis, members can act as lookouts — or in the jargon of the TUC, watchdogs — and help safety reps identify hazards. This has the further advantage of involving members directly in health and safety activities. Any complaints should be dealt with through an agreed procedure, which must be clearly outlined in the employer's safety-policy statement. Unless the problem requires immediate action it is sensible to follow up any verbal request with a written report to the employer. Where a complaint cannot be resolved then use should be made of the existing industrial relations machinery to reach an agreement.

What Facilities Do Safety Representatives Need?

To do their job efficiently safety reps need an office and facilities for handling paperwork, dealing with members, consulting health and safety specialists, and so on. There is nothing in the Regulations that says employers should provide these facilities, but it is far easier to sort out a problem when the paperwork is readily accessible, that is to say in a filing cabinet rather than on the floor, and information sources, like HSE Codes of Practice, are at hand. So the TUC suggest a basic shopping list of facilities which can be negotiated; these include:

- a room, desk and typewriter;
- a filing cabinet;
- duplicating facilities;
- use of internal and external telephone and post;
- a room for consulting and reporting back to members;
- use of notice boards.

Sources of Information

As a matter of course, safety reps should know how and where to find information. The Regulations give them the right to inspect documents and to receive information from their employer. The

HSC Code of Practice suggests the sort of information which should be given:

- plans and performance of the undertaking relating to safety;
- technical information about hazards and safety precautions for equipment, substances, machinery and systems of work;
- accident, dangerous occurrences and notifiable industrial diseases statistics;
- details of any changes affecting health and safety;
- results of measurements and tests;
- information from manufacturers, importers or suppliers of articles or substances used at work, or proposed to be used.

In addition, the employer has a legal duty under section 2(2(c)) of the Health and Safety at Work Act to provide information on all potential hazards within the workplace, and details of health and safety legislation, Codes of Practice and HSE publications relevant to the workplace. For instance, safety reps responsible for laboratories should have access to a copy of the Code of Practice for the Prevention of Infection in Clinical Laboratories and Post-Mortem Rooms. Similarly, the HSC publications on lifting and on disposal of hospital waste should be readily available.

Again, before approaching management, safety reps will want to know how serious or dangerous a particular hazard may be. Judgments will have to be made to answer the questions:

- What is a reasonable temperature?
- What is overcrowding?
- How many first-aid boxes should there be?

To answer these it is necessary to know where to find information on suitable standards by which to measure the seriousness of these hazards. Some of the common sources of standards are now listed.

HSE Guidance Notes

These notes are published under five subject headings; General, Plant and Machinery, Environmental Hygiene, Chemical Safety, and Medical.

HSE Booklets

These give advice on the application of regulations made under the Health and Safety at Work Act.

HSW Booklets

The Health and Safety at Work Booklets are designed to give up-to-date facts and advice about the best practices in health and safety in the workplace.

The Factories Act 1961

Although the requirements here apply to factories, the Act provides a guide to the minimum standards acceptable to the Health and Safety Inspectorate.

The Offices, Shops and Railway Premises Act 1963

Again, the requirements here are not directly relevant but constitute a guide to the minimum standards acceptable to the Health and Safety Inspectorate.

Department of Health and Social Security Periodicals and Series

The DHSS issue the following publications:

- *Health Service Estate* (quarterly);
- *Current Literature on Health Services* (monthly);
- *Health Equipment Information*;
- *Hazard Warning Notices*;
- *Engineering Data Sheets*.

All these publications are directly relevant to work in the health services, so get management to provide copies of them.

As well as trying to find out information themselves, safety reps have the right to receive information from inspectors, in accordance with section 28(8) of the Health and Safety at Work Act, following visits to the workplace.

Besides legal assistance for accidents at work, many unions now provide their safety reps with information about specific hazards as

well as useful handbooks on their rights and details of relevant
health and safety legislation. Some unions have got to the stage
where they have appointed national officers with responsibility for
health and safety, and part of their job is providing information to
safety reps. For example, the GMBATU have a national health
and safety officer but also regional health and safety officers who
are able to visit workplaces and advise members. Again these
officials are able to provide information to safety reps. However,
limited resources have meant that many of the smaller unions are
not able to give a similar service. In this situation the TUC is able
to help by providing an information service for all affiliated
unions. Requests for assistance should go through the branch and
full-time official.

Tackling Problems

Having said a great deal about the Health and Safety at Work Act
and the Safety Representatives and Safety Committees Regulations, we look next at how to use them to improve working
conditions, starting from the very beginning.

Join a union

Obviously, the first step is for everyone in the hospital to join a
recognised and independent health service union like NUPE,
GMBATU or COHSE. Clearly, it is better to get everyone into
the same union, otherwise there will be the age-old problem of
inter-union rivalry. Try to establish a closed shop; the strength of
the union very much depends on everyone joining.

Elect safety reps

Of course, just joining the union will not improve things; the next
step is to elect safety reps for each part of the hospital. As soon as
possible after this they should attend a TUC training course. As
we said earlier, safety reps are allowed time off with pay for
training.

Pick a problem

There will be no shortage of problems facing members, so pick one which is of most concern to them. For instance, suppose members in the hospital laundry have been complaining about high temperatures, especially in the summer, then the first thing to do is find out whether there is a hazard or not. Conduct a survey of members to check if:

- anyone feels tired, weak or sick;
- anyone has felt giddy or faint;
- the laundry is hot and humid.

If the answer is yes to any of these questions, the next step is to:

Read up on the problem

Consult Chapter 5 and any other available literature on temperature and humidity, see bibliography. In table 5.1 we give the Chartered Institute of Building Services 'Comfort Scale' showing acceptable temperatures for different types of work. Probably a temperature of around 12°C is best as most laundry work can be described as moderately heavy. And on page 95 we suggest indoor humidity levels should be kept to between 40 and 75 per cent. Having found suitable standards then:

Approach management

Having satisfied yourself that there is probably a health and safety problem, approach management. Ask for temperature measurements to be made in different parts of the laundry throughout the day. At the same time get management to measure the humidity levels. Then compare these observations with the standards given in the previous step, that is, 12°C and 40 to 75 per cent humidity levels. If this confirms that there is a problem then the best strategy is to improve ventilation and install a humidifier; see Chapter 5.

No action

Often, management dismisses the problems as unimportant or complains that money is not available to make improvements. In either case, it is best to call in your full-time union official for advice and assistance. Of course, there is no guarantee that your union official is going to be any more successful.

Union response

If management are unwilling to improve conditions there are several courses of action available, as follows.

- Call in an HSE inspector — but they will come only if the matter cannot be dealt with through existing procedures..
- Industrial action, or the prospect of it, might 'persuade' management to be more sympathetic.
- Tell the local press, MP and Community Health Council.

Remember, the strength of the union and the success of safety reps very much depends on involving members. So keep them informed at every stage because they will decide whether the solution is satisfactory; it will be up to them to take action if it is not.

SAFETY COMMITTEE

The Safety Representatives and Safety Committees Regulations 1978 provide for the setting up of a safety committee where at least two safety reps ask that one be set up. But experience has shown that too many of these tend to be 'tea and biscuits' committees where agendas are cluttered up with trivia and decision making is always put off. So it is vital to decide at the outset the role of the committee. To begin with, complaints made by safety reps should be dealt with through an agreed health and safety procedure and not channelled through the committee; then the guidance notes issued with the Regulations give some idea of what topics should be dealt with by the committee, namely:

- consideration of the workplace safety policy;
- study of the accident and notifiable-diseases statistics so that your employer knows of any unsafe or unhealthy conditions or practices;
- consideration of new legislation or reports relevant to the workplace;

- action on health and safety problems affecting the whole workplace;
- effectiveness of health and safety publicity in the workplace;
- effectiveness of safety training.

But this list is not final; it is a matter of negotiation at local level what each safety committee actually does. The guidance notes merely list the basic functions that a safety committee could carry out.

To stop the safety committee simply turning into a 'tea party' safety reps should set up their own committee where they decide what items they want on the safety committee agenda, agree their priorities, discuss the arguments that will be used and choose who will speak on each issue. By organising this kind of pre-meeting safety reps will make the safety committee more effective. It will also bring together all recognised unions in the workplace and make them that much more effective.

Now, the committee is made up of management and union representatives. The management side will obviously be unwilling to accept many of the unions' suggestions for improving safety, generally on the grounds of cost and whether the improvements are really necessary. On the other hand, safety reps will be pushing for improvement in all levels of safety. But what happens if recommendations are ignored by management? A safety committee has no legal power to force management to take up its suggestions. In practice, when this happens safety reps can either ignore the safety committee or refer outstanding issues to shop stewards so that they can be dealt with through the established collective bargaining procedures.

SAFETY POLICIES

We have already said a lot about the work of safety reps and something about the role of safety committees. We need now to look at safety policies, which are very important in so far as they express the employer's commitment to providing a safe workplace. The HSE say they should:

- recognise the importance of health and safety;
- ensure that responsibilities, both legal and managerial, are

clearly defined and understood throughout the organisation;
- establish the arrangements for dealing with the health and safety needs of the various activities carried out;
- monitor and review progress at regular intervals.

In the case of the NHS it is impossible to have a single policy which would apply to all workplaces, because of the size of the organisation and variety of work. In fact, the HSE suggest that the policy should be dealt with in three parts, as follows:

General. This is the overall policy of the Authority or Health Board and should include:

- a basic declaration to provide safe and healthy working conditions;
- an outline of those in management who have responsibility for health and safety;
- details on training, consultation, monitoring and arrangements for implementing DHSS recommendations on equipment and buildings.

Specialist. This is the policy of a District Nursing Officer, District Works Officer and other equivalent posts and should include:

- an indication of how the relevant parts of the general policy will be put into action;
- a chart or similar means showing those in management with responsibility for health and safety, an indication of how information will be given and the names of experts like the radiation protection officer;
- arrangements for consultation, training and the identification of hazards and means of controlling them.

Unit. This is the policy which most workers will have direct contact with, as it refers to the local district hospital, mental handicap hospital and similar health service establishments. Basically, it should include, like the specialist policy:

- an indication of how the relevant parts of the general policy will be implemented;

- details of those with responsibility for implementing health and safety measures, an indication of how information will be given and guidance on the role of specialist services like the occupational health service and fire prevention officer;
- arrangements for consultation, for monitoring performance, and for dealing with the safety of the general public, contractors and workers in other departments who may be affected by work in a particular department; also, finally, details of the hazards in each department and how they should be controlled.

We have set out only the broad details of each policy; more will be found in an HSC publication *Safety Policies in the Health Services*.

An effective safety policy is an important weapon in the battle for safer and healthier working conditions. It is therefore important to see that the policy leads to improvements. This can be done by monitoring, the HSC say,

- all accident and ill-health statistics;
- all near misses and dangerous occurrences;
- whether legal standards and codes of practice are met;
- the extent to which long-term objectives are met and the time taken to agree them;
- whether the measures proposed in each policy statement are carried out.

This list is not exhaustive, and other ways may be found. These are likely to depend on the type of hazard, for instance regular monitoring of waste anaesthetic gases in operating theatres.

NOTICES AND CROWN IMMUNITY

The powers of the Health and Safety inspectors are set out in sections 21 to 25 of the Health and Safety at Work Act. These give inspectors the authority to issue improvement and prohibition notices. An improvement notice tells the employer what he must do to improve the health, safety or welfare of a particular part of his workplace and ignoring it is a criminal offence. Similarly, a prohibition notice is served wherever there is a serious risk of injury. If the risk is high then the notice can stop a particular job or close down a department but if the risk is less serious then the notice will give a time limit during which the inspector's recommendations must be carried out.

Sections 33 to 42 deal with the powers of prosecution for failing to comply with the Act or notices served by an inspector. It is here that exemption from these legal duties is given to the health service on the grounds that it is, in legal terms, 'the Crown' and cannot prosecute itself. Of course, if the health service were a model employer setting high standards for private employers to emulate there would be no problem. But it is clear that this is not the case. In fact, as far back as 1968 the Tunbridge Committee, set up to look into health and safety standards in hospitals, commented:

> For too long the hospital service has failed to give a lead to others in the care of staff that one would expect from an employer of well over half a million people and from an organisation devoted to the care of the sick. It is time it started to give that lead.

The Committee went further and said:

> The National Health Service has paid some attention to 40 per cent of its staff which comprises of nurses, but the rest — domestics, cleaners, porters and catering staff — have been sadly neglected.

However, in 1978 the HSE did give inspectors the power to issue a new form of notice against Crown employers. The notice, called the Crown notice, is much the same as improvement and prohibition notices except that it has no force in law. It has two uses, though: first it gives inspectors a means for exerting pressure on an employer to improve safety standards, and second, if unions are aware of what the inspector has recommended then they can also put pressure on the employer. However, there appears to be some reluctance on the part of inspectors to use Crown notices. In 1980 about 15,000 improvement and prohibition notices were issued whereas only 30 to 40 Crown notices were issued in the same period (see Chapter 9).

Table 8.1   Provision of OH services in 1980 (percentages in brackets indicate where provision is made for workers outside the NHS)

	Single hospitals	Group of hospitals	District	Health Authority
OH services				
(%)	1.43	N/A	29.6	34.5
	(0.2)	(N/A)	(7.2)	(18.5)

OCCUPATIONAL HEALTH SERVICE

Little attention has been paid to the occupational health problems of health workers. The traditional role of hospitals has been the treatment of ill health rather than its prevention. All too often, this has meant health authorities overlooking the need of occupational health (OH) services for their staff. As a result, hospital workers have sought advice from one another, these 'corridor consultations' making the demand for OH services.

The inadequacy of the existing provision can be seen from a study by the Employment Medical Advisory Service (EMAS) of health service OH services (table 8.1).

Even the percentages in the table are misleading: only 28 per cent had a doctor in charge, and only 3 per cent of these were full time. Again, only one in seven doctors actually held a recognised OH qualification, while just over one in three nurses in charge of OH services had a specialist qualification.

In 1979 the Deputy Director of EMAS, Dr E.S. Blackadder, in an article in the *Royal Society of Health Journal* on OH service provision in the NHS, complained that 'It is, therefore, disappointing that so little progress appears to have been made in providing an Occupational Health Service staffed by adequately trained doctors and nurses for the NHS.'

Despite this gloomy picture, opinion in favour of OH services for health workers is gathering momentum. Even the DHSS has issued a draft Circular and Notes of Guidance on the development of OH services, and the HSC has set up the Industry Advisory Committee for the Health Service, one of whose priorities has been the establishment of a working party to draft guidance on OH services for the NHS. We had better not get carried away with enthusiasm over these developments, since after all it is fifteen years since the Tunbridge Committee report *The Care of the Health of Hospital Staff* first recommended the setting up of OH services.

In the remainder of this chapter we look at what an OH department does and who works in it.

What Is the Role of an Occupational Health Service?

Most accidents and occupational diseases are certainly avoidable if the right steps are taken. This seems obvious, but what is the best way of achieving it? In this chapter, we argue that the setting up of an occupational health service is one way of making the workplace safer. Such an OH service would have these functions:

- prevention;
- pre-employment screening;
- immunisation;
- rehabilitation;
- counselling;
- health education;
- health records;
- treatment;
- staff welfare

We now look at each of these in turn to see what is required.

Prevention

Of the functions of an OH service the most important is the prevention of accidents and ill health. This means that all hazards in the workplace have to be identified. To do this requires regular inspections of places like kitchens, laundries and laboratories; it also requires the monitoring of absences due to accidents and other causes, which includes environmental and biological monitoring in addition to the examination of health records. Bedford

General Hospital's OH department soon found out the value of regular inspections after a survey of their catering department showed the standards of hygiene to be below those demanded in industry.

The hazards having been found, it is obviously necessary to find ways of preventing them, and this will include giving advice on the planning and design of new buildings, equipment and work practices as well as guidance in statutory requirements. Again the experience of Bedford General's OH department is worth drawing on. The hospital built their catering building without first consulting the OH department about the design, with the result that the staff rest room had no daylight, toilet facilities were unsatisfactory, showers were not provided for catering staff, ventilation in the kitchens was inadequate and, believe it or not, the floor did not slope towards the drains.

Pre-employment screening

Most jobs don't require a pre-employment medical; it is only for jobs which are known to be dangerous, like deep-sea diving, or which call for very expensive training, like being an airline pilot, that they are insisted upon. However, one of the functions of an OH service is to organise pre-employment screening. There are several reasons for doing this, namely to find the following.

- Those whose health could be put at risk by their job. We argue in Chapter 6, on the subject of stress, that working with the terminally ill or with the seriously ill in an intensive-care unit is very stressful, so it is common sense to identify those most susceptible to stress and let them work in other wards.
- Workers with special health problems who may need to be under observation like diabetics or the disabled.
- Those with illnesses requiring treatment. Normally, these would be referred to their own doctor.
- Whether an applicant is fit to do a particular job. However, this is much more controversial because it gives the employer the chance of turning down an applicant on grounds of ill health rather than trying to find alternative work for them. Again, Bedford General OH department found very few instances of workers unfit for employment on medical grounds. Always

insist that your employer makes every effort to find alternative work before turning down an applicant.

There is no need to give a full medical to each applicant: a simple health questionnaire with a guarantee of confidentiality is good enough. If any health problems are identified by the questionnaire, an interview with the occupational health nurse is usually sufficient. But a small minority of cases, as little as two in a hundred, normally require a physical examination.

Immunisation programme

Infectious diseases are a major risk in hospitals so an immunisation programme is essential, and should be the responsibility of the OH service who can keep complete records of those vaccinated. Some of the diseases that call for immunisation include the following.

Tuberculosis. Although the number of people with TB has fallen it is still possible to contract the disease. A case may be admitted to hospital and it will be several days before the disease is diagnosed; meanwhile doctors, nurses and domestics will have had regular contact with the patient. Other workers like radiographers may also come into contact with the patient, so everyone should be offered protection.

Tetanus. Since there are few side effects with this vaccine everyone should be encouraged to accept it.

Polio. Again, the likelihood of contracting this disease is rare but outbreaks do occur, so everyone needs protection. Remember, it was not so long ago that with banner headlines newspapers were telling the tragic story of polio striking down a footballer at the peak of his career, leaving him a cripple in an iron lung.

Rubella. Protection should be given to all workers in the maternity and paediatric departments, especially women of childbearing age. But rubella vaccine need be given only to those who have no natural protection against the disease; a simple test can determine this. Women who contract rubella within the first three months of pregnancy invariably give birth to a deaf, dumb and blind baby, so immunity against the disease is vital.

Typhoid.   As a matter of course laundry workers and others who handle soiled linen should be offered protection.

Flu.   Again, all workers should be offered protection against this debilitating illness.

It is arguable whether immunisation against diphtheria and smallpox are worth having since outbreaks of diphtheria are virtually unknown and, with the exception of the outbreak at Birmingham University Medical School in 1978, smallpox has been eradicated. Equally, it is now likely that more workers will be allergic to the vaccination than would actually contract smallpox. Nevertheless, laboratory workers handling these germs must be vaccinated.

Although immunisation should remain voluntary, workers should be encouraged to participate. Once again, the experience of Bedford General's OH department illustrates the importance of an immunisation programme. A patient with rubella was admitted to one of the wards, and the sister was able to confirm with the OH department that all her staff were protected.

Rehabilitation

We argue in this chapter that counselling is an essential function of an OH service. So it seems obvious that after accidents or absence because of long-term sickness the OH service should provide a counselling service to find out what special provisions, if any, an individual may need to adjust to their job. For instance, a nurse with a back injury should not be asked to work in a geriatric ward where lifting patients is a regular part of the job; instead alternative work should be offered. Of course, some employers would see this as the ideal opportunity to transfer, downgrade or make redundant a worker in this situation. Why should this be allowed to happen? After all, accidents usually happen because workplaces are not designed with safety in mind. So alternative employment or retraining has got to be the answer.

Counselling

While many accidents are caused by the conditions at work, for instance poor lighting, lack of lifting aids and so on, there are also other reasons for them. Workers can have domestic problems which they bring to work, poor health like depression, or personality clashes with colleagues at work, all of which may lead to mistakes and, eventually, to accidents at work. Quite clearly, one of the functions of an OH service is to help people with problems like these, and this is best done by providing an occupational health counselling service available to everyone. Basically, the counselling would set out to identify those factors which are contributing to a worker's ill health and provide suitable advice and help. Of course, where there is a medical problem the individual should be sent to their own doctor.

Health education

There is no doubt that smoking, drinking, lack of exercise and being overweight can lead to poor health among workers. Very little can be done to improve the diet of most workers simply because they can't afford the better foods like steaks and so on, although health education can warn against excessive intake of fatty and overcooked foods. But something can be done about smoking, drinking and lack of sufficient exercise. Although no government control is exercised over the tobacco and drink industries (by this we mean that the government is unwilling to stop them advertising cigarettes and beer), we feel that everyone should be discouraged from smoking, drinking in excess and jogging — walking is actually much better for you. It is here that the OH service has a useful role in promoting greater awareness of these health problems. In addition, there is no reason why they should not also be involved in encouraging screening for breast and cervical cancer, both of which respond to treatment if caught early enough.

Health records

As we argue throughout this chapter, the primary function of an OH service is the prevention of accidents and occupational diseases at work. To do this demands not only inspections of the workplace but also records of the incidence, distribution and control of occupational illnesses and accidents. If, however there is to be agreement on the keeping of health records then a guarantee of complete confidentiality must be given by the employer. In practice this means that no information on any worker is given to the employer without the prior approval in writing of the individual concerned. In their guidelines on an OH service the HSE suggest that only the occupational doctor or nurse needs to have access to these records and some of the information that might be kept could include:

- initial and subsequent health questionnaire, interview, examination and screening test results;
- relevant medical and occupational history, smoking habits, disabilities and handicaps;
- general health care and counselling;
- injuries from occupational and non-occupational accidents;
- illnesses at work;
- sickness absences;
- occupational conditions and diseases;
- care and treatment given;
- recommendation and work limitations imposed;
- referrals made to other specialists or agencies;
- correspondence relating to the health of the employee;
- communications between occupational health staff and others, including written reports.

To ensure complete confidentiality none of this documentation should leave the OH department.

Treatment

It is not the function of an OH service to give a 24-hour comprehensive medical service for workers but simply to provide first aid and emergency treatment only. Naturally, anyone who is feeling sick can be seen but this should only be emergency treatment until they can visit their own doctor. If an accident happens, treatment should be given by casualty, and details of the incident passed to the OH service for their records. Besides treating minor illnesses and injuries the OH service has an important part to play in the training of first aiders and in the supervision of statutory first-aid regulations. Finally, one advantage of providing this kind of cover is in the identification of possible health hazards by analysing details of all cases referred to the OH service for treatment.

Staff welfare

All too often the facilities for workers like toilets and canteens are totally unsatisfactory, as the experience of Bedford General Hospital has shown. Again, this is an area where the experience of the OH service has a role to play. Their expertise can be put to good use in seeing that statutory requirements are in fact met, and that welfare provisions meet the needs of the workplace.

The Team Approach

Detecting, controlling and preventing accidents and ill health at work cannot be seen as the sole responsibility of the safety officer. In fact, it should be the function of what we call an 'occupational health team', which would comprise:

- occupational health doctor;
- occupational health nurse;
- occupational hygienist;
- safety officer.

Each member of the team brings a particular skill that can be utilised when dealing with a hazard. For instance, pollution of operating theatres and anterooms by waste anaesthetic gases is a serious problem calling for action from the whole team. Regular monitoring of anaesthetic gas levels and checking the effectiveness of ventilation would be done by the occupational hygienist, installation of scavenging systems for removal of waste gases would be for the safety officer to deal with, while, finally, health checks of operating theatre staff would be the function of the occupational health doctor or nurse. This example clearly demonstrates the need for a team approach and relies upon close co-operation between all the members. Let us look, in more detail, at each member of this team.

Occupational Health Doctors and Nurses

Medical staff running this service should have the proper training: doctors and nurses should possess specialist occupational health qualifications. This seems obvious, but an EMAS survey, done in 1976, showed that only 17½ per cent of doctors dealing with occupational health services held a specialist qualification while for nurses it was 19 per cent. Yet courses are available. So it is essential to check that medical staff appointed to an OH service actually hold appropriate qualifications. (We looked at the work done by occupational health staff at the beginning of this chapter.)

Occupational Hygienist

The role of the occupational hygienist is the recognition, evaluation and control of environmental hazards which cause sickness or affect the general health and well being of workers. As well as using her skills to monitor the environment for suspected hazards the hygienist should be available to give advice on possible health problems related to new systems of work or new medical procedures that may be introduced into the hospital.

Like the safety officer, the hygienist will frequently be called upon to give advice about some problem or other. So it is important that she remains independent of management and able to give impartial advice on the full range of options available to deal with the suspected hazard. For example, if asked to give advice on how to deal with cleaning agents which are causing dermatitis the hygienist should be willing to set out all the choices. These will probably include advice on skin care, the use of alternative cleaning products and the use of rubber gloves.

Again, the person holding this post should be expected to hold the specialist qualifications in occupational hygiene that are available.

Safety Officer

Clearly, the safety officer has a key role to play in identifying, controlling and eliminating hazards. Of these the prevention of hazards must be the most important. This means recognising them through regular surveys of the workplace, through investigating dangerous occurrences and accidents and, finally, through the examination of plans for any proposed new buildings and procedures. In addition, the safety officer should be expected to have a thorough grasp of all relevant health and safety law and other requirements. Part of his function will also be to provide information on all possible hazards in the workplace. To fulfil this very important function we would expect him to set up a comprehensive health and safety library, available to all safety reps.

Finally, employers have a duty under the Health and Safety at Work Act to provide safety training. Of course, we expect all safety reps to take the basic ten-day TUC course, but the employer should give training on specialist problems in his workplace. So the safety officer can be expected to arrange for, and possibly carry out, these training programmes. For example, in Chapter 7 we look at the current problem of violence to staff. Obviously, this is of only limited interest to most safety reps and is not a hazard dealt with on the basic ten-day TUC course. It would be the responsibility of the employer to see that the safety officer arranges suitable training on this matter.

As in the case of the other members of the occupational health team, we stress the importance of checking that the safety officer is qualified, and not the fire officer doubling up.

The Independence of the OH Service

In their report, *The Care of the Health of Hospital Staff*, the Tunbridge Committee stressed that the OH service should be independent of the usual hospital management structure. In our view, this can best be done by making the occupational health team accountable to the Hospital Management Committee through an Occupational Health Committee. To be effective, committee membership should be as compact as possible, and there should be at least equal representation of management and union. The OH doctor and nurse, hygienist and safety officer should be ex-officio members and the position of chair should alternate between management and union. Where a safety committee exists, the ex-officio members of the OH committee should, in our view, be invited to attend.

It is important to establish at the outset what the role of the OH committee is to be. So matters which are the responsibility of the safety committee should not be dealt with (see Chapter 8).

Instead, the committee should confine its role to consideration of those functions listed at the beginning of this section (prevention, pre-employment screening, and so on) as well as reports of the OH team.

In this section we have set out our views on how to establish an effective OH service for health service workers. Those who want to know more should read the booklet *Workplace Health and Safety Services* which gives the TUC's views on this subject. Remember, once an OH service is in operation the best way of measuring its effectiveness is to see whether there is a fall in the rate of occupational accidents and illnesses and whether people use it.

REFERENCES

Association of Scientific, Technical and Managerial Staffs (1982). *Comments on DHSS Draft Health Notice*, Occupational Health Services in the NHS. ASTMS, London

Bedford General Hospital Occupational Health Service (1975). *7th and Final Report*. North Bedfordshire Health Authority, 3 Kimbolton Road, Bedford, MK40 2NU

E.S. Blackadder (1979). Occupational health services for NHS staff. *R. Soc. Health J.* **4**. 137–9

Employers' occupational health service and the group schemes. Industrial relations review and report. *Health and Safety Information Bulletin* No. 77 (1982)

J.P. Gracie (1982). Health surveillance in industry. *Occupational Health in Ontario*, **3**, 20–32

R. Lewy (1981). Prevention strategies in hospital occupational medicine. *J. occup. Med.*, **23**, 109–11

J.A. Lunn (1976). *The Health of Staff in Hospitals*. Heinemann Medical Books, London, chh. 2–4

National Union of Public Employees (1978). *Health and Safety at Work*. NUPE, London

Trades Union Congress (1980). *Workplace Health and Safety Services: TUC Proposals For an Integrated Approach*. TUC, London

9. The Future

There is no doubt that the Health and Safety at Work Act is an important piece of legislation. It brought within the scope of the law eight million workers not previously covered by any safety legislation including nearly a million health service workers. For them safety had been dealt with as a collective bargaining issue, with the end result usually a compromise on the part of workers.

One example illustrates the sort of problems hospital workers faced before the Act. Sid, a laundry worker, collapsed from heat exhaustion in the hospital laundry. Despite requests from the staff nothing had been done to improve ventilation in the laundry; management were not prepared to spend money on it. The workers in the laundry decided to strike until fans and extractors were installed. However, they eventually had to settle for a compromise: frequent rest periods outside the main laundry room.

The situation has improved to some extent since the Act came into operation. To begin with unions have the legal right to appoint or elect safety reps who can inspect the workplace and represent the workers' interests in terms of health and safety matters. These important rights reflect the fact that employers had consistently failed to take safety as seriously as production. They also recognise the important role of unions in dealing with workers' ill health and accidents, and that they could no longer be denied the right to participate in decisions affecting the health and safety of their members.

Of course, to be effective safety reps need access to information from all sources. In the past, the employer's obligation to provide this was fulfilled by posting abstracts from the Factories Act 1961 and various regulations under it, most of which were piecemeal and limited in scope. In practice, this meant little information was actually made available to safety reps in the health services. The Act changed all this by requiring employers to provide safety reps with as much information as is necessary for them to carry out their duties.

Apart from the general duties imposed on employers and manufacturers, the Act encourages a closer relationship between workers and the HSE inspectors. Before 1974, Factory Inspectors were not allowed to inform workers about the risks they might face at work. For instance, if an inspector were to monitor the levels of, say, formaldehyde, he was forbidden to pass his results to the workers. But this has changed with the passage of the Act. Workers can now expect to be given a wide range of information including details of any improvement or prohibition notices served, although it is still left to discretion of the individual inspector to decide what information he considers 'necessary' to keep workers 'adequately' informed.

LIMITS OF THE ACT

It is not much use having laws if all employers do is ignore them. Enforcing safety law is the responsibility of HSE inspectors of which there are about 830 available to visit 750,000 workplaces. About half their time is actually spent visiting. In practice, this means bad workplaces receive a visit once every three years whereas others will see an inspector only once in a decade. The inspectorate plan to complete the first rounds of inspection of health service workplaces by 1983. As we argue later in this chapter, the inability of the inspectors to visit workplaces regularly means that effective trade union organisation is the only practical way of dealing with safety.

On top of all this, inspectors face another problem, namely the exclusion of the health services from the provision in the Act enabling the prosecution of employers failing to comply with the law. This all comes about, as we saw in Chapter 8, because the NHS is the Crown in legal terms and cannot be prosecuted. In practice, this has meant that health authorities which do not comply with recommendations of an inspector, say, to provide suitable containers for sharps cannot be fined. However, inspectors can issue Crown improvement or prohibition notices, although they have no force in law.

Clearly, this state of affairs is unsatisfactory. HSE statistics show the reluctance of inspectors to issue Crown notices without legal backing: only about 40 were served in the health services in 1980 whereas 15,000 were served on private industry. Health service unions like COHSE, NALGO and NUPE want to change this, and have taken it up with successive governments. There appears to be little sympathy for this proposal from Jim Hammer, Her Majesty's Chief Inspector of Factories. In an interview published in April 1982 in the monthly journal *Safety*, he said in reply to a question about Crown immunity:

> ... I entirely understand the views of those who say why should major employers be exempt from prosecution.
>
> I'm much more of a pragmatist on this and I tend to look at the set-up and ask how often we actually had to back off and accept conditions we were unhappy with which we could have changed if we had been able to prosecute. I can't see that there are many such circumstances.
>
> We have issued Crown notices with the threat that if they don't comply it would end up at top levels of the DHSS. Forty-six Crown notices on hospitals for instance in two and a half years is not many but it just shows how persuasive we are. (Laughter from audience.)

On the same page in *Safety*, the Factory Inspectorate report issuing 1,362 notices immediately prohibiting a process, and a further 223 deferring prohibition. In all 4,385 improvement notices were issued. As for local authorities, 6,223 improvement notices were issued, 779 immediate prohibition notices and 224 deferred prohibition notices. Allowing for the fact that it is not straightforward to draw comparisons between different industries we find it difficult to believe that the health services are so much safer that only 46 Crown notices were needed in over two and a half years.

A more plausible explanation for the small number of Crown notices may be the one given (in *Safety*, March 1982) by Pat Woodcock, the HSE official with overall responsibility for enforcing safety in the Health Services. He believes there are probably two reasons for this: 'One is our [the HSE's] lack of power to ensure that failure to comply with a notice would end up in a court of law. The other is the fact that we are still working through the first round of visits to health service premises.' Certainly there are grounds, as we have said, for removing Crown immunity so that notices having legal backing and for providing more inspectors to visit workplaces and police the law.

Apart from the fact that health authorities cannot be fined, non-Crown employers caught breaking the law usually escape with a token fine as the following list shows:

Offence	Average fine
Carcinogens	£233
Asbestos	£210
Toxic substances	£124
Biological hazards	N/A
Storage of flammable substances	£189
Dangerous materials	£250

In 1980 the average fine was only £170 even though magistrates have the authority to fine offenders up to a maximum of £1,000. One example illustrates clearly the paltry fines magistrates impose, even when workers are killed. Gerry was taking measurements inside a ten-foot deep drainage trench when the sides collapsed crushing him. In spite of the fact that the company admitted negligence the defence counsel asked for leniency on the grounds that 'this tragic event must be borne by the company morally for a substantial time to come'. The magistrates fined the company £250 although the Factory Inspector had pressed for the maximum penalty under the regulations of £1,000. In fact, it is very rare for magistrates actually to fine an employer the maximum penalty even when he is negligent. So the price of life is less than £1,000.

Although many people argue that compensation claims are sufficient incentive for employers to provide comfortable, safe and healthy workplaces, we don't agree. Certainly, available evidence

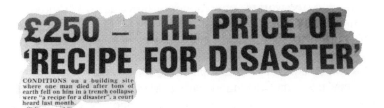

£250 – THE PRICE OF 'RECIPE FOR DISASTER'

CONDITIONS on a building site where one man died after tons of earth fell on him in a trench collapse were "a recipe for a disaster", a court heard last month.

Fines: only £250 for Gerry's death.

does not support this view and we would argue that fines should be much higher; perhaps even the threat of jail would not be amiss.

It may be worth while comparing the value of life against the fines imposed on an employer when someone is killed. The National Radiological Protection Board has recently made calculations based on the cost of shortening a life in terms of loss of output, medical costs and so on, and also on what workers are willing to pay for a decrease in risk on the sum they would accept as compensation for an increase in risk; the result of these calculations was that life has a value in the range of £100,000 to £2½ million. Compare this with a trivial fine of £250 for negligently allowing the death of an employee, and the inescapable conclusion must be that penalties for breaking safety laws are too low. So not only should Crown immunities be removed; penalties for breaking the law must be much tougher.

WHAT NEXT?

Although the Health and Safety at Work Act has undoubtedly secured some improvements, we would argue that there is still scope for more change. In particular, we think the time has come to give safety reps the right to stop the job before accidents happen. Remember Sid, who collapsed from heat exhaustion? Everyone knew that the temperature and humidity were far too high in the laundry yet the employer did nothing. Such incidents could effectively be dealt with if safety reps were able to stop the job; employers would then be much more willing to listen to them.

In fact, the right to stop the job has already been given to safety reps in Sweden and Canada. Statistics from the Swedish National Board of Occupational Health and Safety show that in 1974, when the right to stop working operations was introduced, 52 shutdowns occurred. In 1975 this rose to 94 and, in 1976, shutdowns reached 136, but the following year the figure fell to 97, reflecting the fact that some employers were probably anticipating what their safety reps might do. Jobs were shut down for a variety of reasons, ranging from the closing down of a factory until dangerous machinery had been replaced to the temporary closure of a psychiatric hospital until the nursing–patient ratio was substantially improved.

Of course, we anticipate that most employers will reject this proposal out of hand. But so will some trade unionists. They will argue that it is wrong to give safety reps a power which is not subject to the usual control of shop meetings and consultation with full-time officials. We don't agree: safety reps should be able to recognise potentially dangerous situations and judge whether work needs to be stopped until an HSE inspector is available to look at the problem

CUTS

Despite protests from the HSC and the TUC, the HSE annual budget was slashed for the three years 1979–81. Staffing levels fell from 4,250 in November 1979 to 3,730 at the end of December 1982. Bill Simpson, the head of the HSC, candidly admitted in the foreword to the 1980–1 HSC Report that many small workplaces without special hazards will not be visited unless there is a complaint or, even worse, an accident. Not only have field inspectors been cut back but staff working on regulations, approved codes and guidance have suffered a similar fate. Inevitably, this has meant that many projects have been either deferred or dropped. But the most disturbing aspect is the fact that the average time between visits to workplaces will be longer — those with bad records will be inspected only every three years compared with every other year in 1977. Perhaps the HSC *Plan of Work 1981–82 and Onwards* sums up the situation very neatly: 'The average length of time between visits to workplaces will be longer than before the passing of the 1974 [HASAW] Act.' Undoubtedly, the first priority must be to reinstate the overall budget to its full 1979 value. As a TUC spokesperson has pointed out at a meeting with the Secretary of State for Employment, the relatively small sum of only £10 million could transform health and safety provision in this country.

FUNDING FOR SAFETY

The lack of financial resources for dealing with health and safety in the NHS is a serious barrier to improvements. The system of financing it since the introduction of cash limits invariably means money spent on safety must come off patient care or staff wages.

In this climate it is not surprising that unions as well as employers find it difficult to allocate part of the budget to health and safety. Clearly, the care of the sick is an immediate and easily recognisable priority whereas worker safety is not. However, why should workers face this choice?

The very nature of increasing demands on the NHS means that there will always be a need for more money to improve the service to patients. That is why we argue that money must be earmarked for health and safety over and above the annual budget for running the NHS. That way the much-needed improvements can be paid for without affecting patient care. No longer would a health authority be faced with the unpalatable choice between, say, providing air conditioning in a hospital laundry and opening an empty ward.

Of course, this begs the question: how much money should be set aside? And how should it be spent? Clearly, a rolling programme of improvements is required since the health services have a legacy of poor working conditions going back over a century in many of our hospitals. As to the future, the mistakes of the past need not be repeated. New hospitals should be built with safety in mind: wards designed to allow the use of lifting aids, operating suites given adequate ventilation and so on. Clearly, consultation needs to take place with safety reps so that the lessons of the past are actually put into practice.

An immediate priority of any health and safety programme within the health services is the establishment of an occupational health service, the cornerstone of any policy of accident and disease prevention. Since cash limits are the order of the day, a programme of accident and disease prevention should appeal to health authorities. It not only saves lives but also money which otherwise might be spent on compensation payments to injured workers.

Of course, spending on health and safety capital projects has a beneficial effect on the economy as a whole since it increases demand for goods and services which, in turn, brings employment. It is good sense to provide safer working conditions for health service workers as well as boosting the nation's economy.

TUC IMPROVEMENTS

The TUC in a recent publication, *Workplace Health and Safety*

Services, has set out ideas on new health and safety legislation. Among the suggestions put forward are:

- an approved Code of Practice obliging employers to provide minimum occupational health and safety services;
- an HSE system for approving and licensing of any services;
- a set of standards to assess the role, functions and qualifications of OHS staff;
- a guide to the mixture of OHS skills needed in any given industry;
- group OHS schemes for small organisations without sufficient money to provide their own.

Behind these proposals is the belief that integrated health and safety services are essential for industry. Instead of working independently, OH nurses and doctors, safety officers and occupational hygienists should offer a team service. Organisations failing to satisfy the minimum standards in the Code of Practice could be subject to improvement notices with the threat of fines for failing to comply. Since very few hospitals have occupational health services these proposals, if they become law, would provide a much-needed driving force to extend them throughout the health service.

THE ROLE OF TRADE UNIONS

As we have pointed out there are limits to protection given by law, partly because there are insufficient inspectors to police it, partly because the fines are pitifully low and partly because magistrates and judges are unwilling to impose the maximum penalties that the law allows. Often, judges offend the spirit of the law by interpreting parts in ways not meant by Parliament and in doing so find in the employer's favour. Perhaps the most common example is the interpretation of the phrase 'reasonably practicable' which is the balance between on the one hand the cost to the employer of safety measures and on the other the risk of injury or disease to workers. For a railwayman this balance meant no compensation. John's leg was crushed when he fell underneath a 60-foot length of rail being lowered by a crane. The judge ruled that slipping was an 'inherent hazard of the job'.

We assume throughout this book that unions are the only organisations capable of ensuring workers have safe, healthy and comfortable working conditions. The law does not solve health and safety problems; it lays down minimum standards which, as we have just seen in John's case, may even be ignored. In this situation unions have an important role to play. After all, health and safety laws, like the Health and Safety at Work Act, do not remove safety issues from the collective-bargaining arena. The minimum standard having been set by the law, it is effectively left to workers and their trade unions to negotiate improvements.

Equally, if health and safety is to be taken seriously then members as well as safety reps should become involved. Make sure that health and safety is on the branch agenda, include safety articles in the branch newsletter, and arrange weekend and evening courses on safety issues. Nearly all the health service unions provide national health and safety services; booklets, posters and information are available to help safety reps tackle problems.

CONCLUSION

Although we have argued throughout this chapter that workers should not rely totally on the law, many of the changes we propose will require legislation. They will then provide both minimum health and safety standards and incentive for employers to provide safer and healthier working conditions. At the same time, unions must see that employers comply with the law, and that improvements are made to existing standards through collective bargaining.

REFERENCES

J. Laurance (1982). *The Hazards of Work. New Society*, 30 September 1982
Surrey Advertiser, 5 March 1982

Glossary

ASTMS	Association of Scientific, Technical and Managerial Sta
COHSE	Confederation of Health Service Employees
DHSS	Department of Health and Social Security
EMAS	Employment Medical Advisory Service
GMBATU	General and Municipal Boilermakers and Allied Trades Union
HASAW	Health and Safety at Work Act etc. 1974
HSC	Health and Safety Commission
HSE	Health and Safety Executive
NALGO	National and Local Government Officers' Association
NIOSH	National Institute of Occupational Safety and Health
NSC	National Staffs Council
NUPE	National Union of Public Employees
SRSC	Safety Representatives and Safety Committees Regulati
TUC	Trades Union Congress

Bibliography

ASBESTOS

A.J.P. Dalton (1979). *Asbestos—Killer Dust*. British Society for Social Responsibility in Science, 9 Poland Street, London W1. A valuable guide to the dangers of asbestos and how to deal with them.

Asbestos in the Urban Environment: *A Manual of Control* (1982). EIA Publications, 9 Ballingham Mansions, Pitt Street, Kensington, London W8. A useful introduction to the hazards of asbestos and what to do with them.

BIOLOGICAL HAZARDS

A. Price, A. Le Serve and D. Parker (1981). *Biological Hazards—The Hidden Threat*. Nelson, London. A guide to biological hazards, the nature of the threat and advice on their detection and control.

CHEMICALS

A.W. Le Serve, C. Vose, C. Wigley, and D. Bennet (1980). *Chemicals, Work and Cancer*. Nelson, London. An explanation of the basic facts on chemical hazards and guidance on their control in the workplace.

GENERAL

TUC (1979). Health and Safety at Work—TUC Guide. Publications Department, TUC, Congress House, Great Russell Street, London WC1. A basic guide on health and safety issues.

P. Kinnersley (1980). *The Hazards of Work—How to Fight Them*.

Pluto Press, Unit 10, Spencer Court, 7 Chalcot Road, London NW1 8LH. A source of information on many hazards including a directory of toxic substances.
Dave Eva and Ron Oswald (1981). *Health and Safety at Work.* Pan, London. A general introduction to health and safety at work written from a trade union point of view.
J.M. Stellman and S.A. Daum (1973). *Work is Dangerous to Your Health.* British Society for Social Responsibility in Science, 9 Poland Street, London W1. An American guide to work hazards, with a list of likely chemical hazards, classified by occupation.

NOISE

TUC (1981). *Noise at Work — A TUC Guide.* Publications Department, TUC, Congress House, Great Russell Street, London WC1. An excellent guide to the problems of noise and what to do about it.

OFFICES

Marianne Craig (1981). *Office Workers' Survival Handbook.* British Society for Social Responsibility in Science, 9 Poland Street, London W1. An invaluable guide to the hazards of working in an office.

REFERENCE

Croner's Health and Safety at Work. Croner Publications Limited, Croner House, 173 Kingston Road, New Malden, Surrey, KT3 3SS. A comprehensive guide to safety law with a bi-monthly amendment service.
Occupational Health and Safety Encyclopaedia (1983). International Labour Office, 96/98 Marsham Street, London SW14 4LY. A valuable although very expensive guide to occupational health and safety.
N.J. Sax (1979). *Dangerous Properties of Industrial Materials,* 4th edition. Again, a useful, although expensive, guide to the hazards and health precautions for most chemicals.

Health and Safety Executive Publications

The following publications are obtainable from Her Majesty's Stationery Office (HMSO), Area Offices of the HSE or some large booksellers.

HSE Guidance Notes. These are published under five subject headings: General, Plant and Machinery, Environmental Hygiene, Chemical Safety and Medical.

Health and Safety at Work Series Booklets. These are a guide to a wide range of specific health and safety problems.

Publications Catalogue 82. This is a catalogue of publications from the Health and Safety Commission and Health and Safety Executive since 1968. All safety reps need a copy of this booklet.

STRESS

N. McDonald and M. Doyle (1981). *The Stresses of Work*. Nelson, London. A very useful introduction to the various social and psychological factors at work and how they can lead to ill health.

Index